FIT HOME TEAM

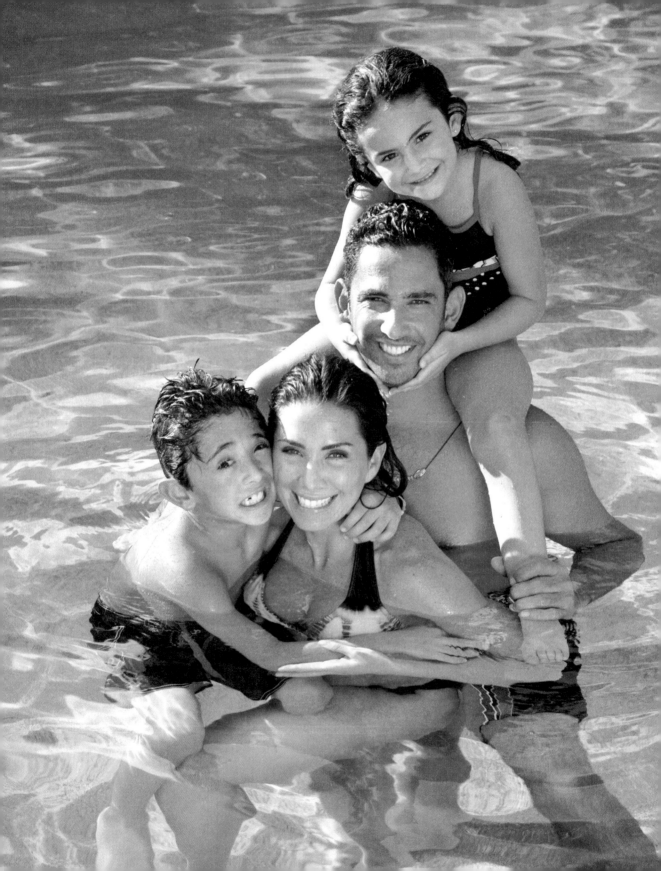

Laura Posada and Jorge Posada

FIT
HOME
TEAM

The Posada Family Guide to Health, Exercise, and Nutrition the Inexpensive and Simple Way

Photography by Chris Fanning

ATRIA BOOKS

NEW YORK LONDON TORONTO SYDNEY

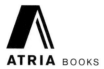

ATRIA BOOKS

A Division of Simon & Schuster, Inc.
1230 Avenue of the Americas
New York, NY 10020

First Atria Books hardcover edition September 2009

ATRIA BOOKS and colophon are trademarks of Simon & Schuster, Inc.

For information about special discounts for bulk purchases,
please contact Simon & Schuster Special Sales at 1-866-506-1949 or
business@simonandschuster.com.

The Simon & Schuster Speakers Bureau can bring authors to
your live event. For more information or to book an event contact
the Simon & Schuster Speakers Bureau at 1-866-248-3049 or
visit our website at www.simonspeakers.com.

Designed by Level C

Manufactured in the United States of America

10 9 8 7 6 5 4 3 2 1

Library of Congress Cataloging-in-Publication Data

Posada, Jorge.
    Fit home team : The Posada family guide to health, exercise, and nutrition the inexpensive and
simple way / Jorge Posada and Laura Posada.
        p.   cm.
    1. Physical fitness. 2. Physical fitness for children.   3. Family recreation.   4. Health.
5. Nutrition. I. Posada, Laura. II. Title.
    GV481.P595 2009
    613.7—dc22   2009013268

ISBN 978-1-4391-0931-1
ISBN 978-1-4391-4961-4 (ebook)

This book is for our children, Jorge Luis and Paulina, the two reasons that we want to be the best that we can possibly be. They are our future and a reflection of us, in the same way that we, too, are mirrors of our own parents.

Both of us come from strong families with marriages that have lasted for more than forty years, fathers who toiled long and hard but always pushed us to be the best; and mothers who always had a warm home-cooked meal waiting for us when we returned from a day at school, or after our games and practices—dicing the onions small enough day after day so that we wouldn't complain. Their love for us was truly endless, just as ours is today for our own.

Thank you, dear parents, for driving us all over Puerto Rico in pursuit of baseball, softball, and volleyball games and every other sporting event in which we decided to participate. It was always a blessing to see that smile on the sideline, even when we struck out or missed a serve. No matter what, we always felt like we were your little champions. We only hope you know that you were also ours.

Contents

The Basics

Healthy Recipes That Never Go Wrong

Foreword

by Bernie Williams
of the New York Yankees

If there is any one thing about baseball that I can say with 100 percent assuredness, it is that the individual is only as good as the rest of his team, and that the group dynamics of any successful team essentially ride on all of the players' ability to collaborate unconditionally. There is a very special strength in the collective force, a sense of empowered unity born directly from the might of a group and its strong determination to prevail victorious. One of the most remarkable things about Jorge Posada, my longtime teammate and close friend, is his ability to apply this lesson about group dynamics to the very place where it matters most—*home.*

Instead of preaching to their son and daughter about the importance of fitness, Jorge and his wife, Laura, themselves participate in their children's experience of exercise—teaching the kids by example and, more important, creating a healthy and productive forum that fosters quality family time. In this way, they not only perpetuate an atmosphere of everyday well-being and vigor but they also instill a sense of personal and collective accountability in the form of fun.

Given the epidemic of obesity among children in the United States, the Posada family approach is one to admire and should also be one to inspire. After all, here is a family who understands firsthand the power of overcoming disease, having endured an eight-year battle with their eldest son's illness, craniosynostosis, a rare condition of the skull. With lionlike courage, the Posadas looked the disease dead in the eye and, with their strong determination, were able to overcome it. But they did not stop there: they consciously decided to make their household one that cherishes wellness above all else, and have since dedicated themselves to this noble pursuit.

In baseball, the catcher is the one who sees everything happening on the field, a vantage point that provides a unique sense of perspective like no other. Jorge Posada, our esteemed catcher and friend, knows this better than anyone else, using his own perspective on life and its tribulations as tools for a greater good. Together with his wife and children, they teach us the power of being strong individuals, and even more so, the unwavering force of their strength as a team.

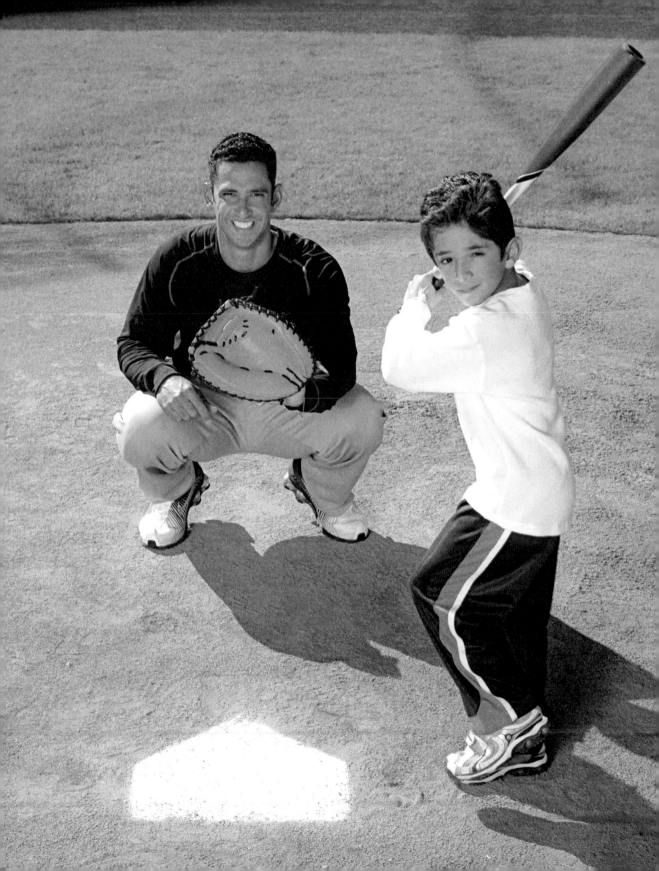

Introduction

When our son was just a tiny little baby, barely able to get himself from point A to point B, we used to (with no regard for our home décor) turn our living room into a sort of crazy funhouse-like obstacle course for him, a microworld of colors, shapes, sizes, challenges, activities, and surprises; each turn heralding a new challenge for our son, and each challenge teaching him something new about mobility, coordination, balance, and many more attributes that would become paramount in our teachings as parents. Little Jorge Luis was entranced by the playful trajectory that we carefully laid out before him, and we, as parents, remained transfixed watching him, at his desire and motivation to get through the game. We saw it as the finest quality time, enriched by the possibility of stimulus, education, and creative activity for our son; plus, it kept *us* on our toes about new and fun ways to entertain him. Those early months and years taught us time and again the invaluable lesson that every moment with one's children is an opportunity to impart some kind of wisdom. That cardinal rule has become the crux of our mission as parents, and so our time together as a family has evolved into a dynamic lifestyle of activities, games, laughs, and delicious food—the building blocks of what great memories are made of and also the building blocks of what strong, healthy kids are made of . . . which is exactly what *Fit Home Team* is all about.

We wrote this book mostly as a testament to our firm belief that our health and our families are perhaps the most important things humans have; and because we believe that, through our experience as this family, we have fine-tuned an interesting balance of health, happiness, and the consistent and collective pursuit of optimal wellness—all through the eyes of our unshakable appreciation for life.

You see, things were not always so rosy: there was a time when we were not sure if our son was going to survive a rare craniofacial condition when he was only a few months old. We can tell you from the bottom of our hearts that putting a baby on an operating table is no easy task. We suffered in uncertainty for many years, and spent many a night not knowing what the next day would bring, if our eldest son would be able to have a normal life, if he would always be afflicted with some kind of pain. But nine years and eight surgeries later, our son prevailed and has fully recovered, growing up into a little warrior of a person—smart, sharp, loving, and strong. We feel it is precisely this blessing that inspires our own gratitude for life, and because of this special miracle, we have dedicated our own lives to raising the healthiest, happiest kids possible. In fact, by having to stay indoors so much in the early phases of his illness, we were forced as parents not only to come up with creative ways to keep him active and entertained but also with the challenge of having to get resourceful about our own workouts. We got ideas from each other, from the various things we had around the house, and even from the physical therapy exercises we picked up for our son as he worked through his recovery to rehabilitate the left side of his body. In this way, what we once considered to be our tragedy transformed itself into our total sense of healing and wellness—for all of us.

Fit Home Team for us represents the power of group effort for the sake of strong lives, and it is our pleasure to bring our passion, experience, and insights to you. With this book we aim to show you how optimal health begins at the root level, with the basic elements of food and fitness at the base of that root—and with your family as the fundamental core of that base. This book is an impassioned invitation to get creative about your approach to total family wellness. It asks you to redefine your conventional sense of fitness, fun, and food by always putting *family* right next to all three words in your mind *and* day-to-day group reality. It aims to inspire you into a new attitude of collective wellness—one based on the principles of resourcefulness, motivation, creativity, love, and positivity.

One of the most disconcerting (not to mention tragic) phenomena we have noticed in this country is the obesity epidemic, especially among children. It is as if the whole nation has been sitting idly by as its children gorge themselves on junk, not knowing that there are healthy, and even tasty, alternatives; not knowing that *exercise* does not have to mean walking a treadmill tediously for an hour or begrudgingly jogging around the block. According to the Office of the Surgeon General, the prevalence of obese adolescents has nearly *tripled* in the last two decades, and overweight adolescents have a 70 percent chance of becoming overweight or obese adults. Worse, the risk factors involved in excess weight include heart disease and related conditions such as high blood pressure and cholesterol, which can lead to more grave problems down the line, including (but not limited to) premature death, type 2 diabetes, hypertension, dyslipidemia, stroke, gallbladder disease, respiratory dysfunction, gout, osteoarthritis, and certain kinds of cancers. Why would anyone tamper with their bodies and invite anything on this horrendous list?

When we begin to understand the concept of wellness as a two-headed beast, we begin to crack the code of optimal health. One of the heads represents fitness and exercise; the other, nutrition. The two work symbiotically, and when mastered in tandem, they can yield life-changing results.

Let's start with one head at a time. We see the pursuit of fitness tracing back to the ancient Greeks, who made it a defining tenet of their culture and philosophy. So why not get with the Greeks, and think of it this way: balance, coordination, strength, and flexibility—these are all words we associate with fitness. But aren't these also words that extend beyond the scope of exercise and fitness into a broader realm of health and wellness? Shouldn't we all aim to be more balanced, coordinated, strong, and flexible—be it on a sports field, in a relationship, or on the job? Today the gamut of exercise is opened up to all kinds of fun-filled possibilities, and so, as parents, our ability to keep our families active has become easier, more dynamic, and more exciting.

We will not only give you tips and suggestions about what kinds of activities to plan for your kids; we will also help you to *rethink* the possibilities, by looking at basic principles, such as the seasons, to help get your juices flowing. We will show you that you don't need much to keep the family active—and that all you really *do* need is a little creativity, determination, and the desire to improve as individuals and as a group.

But, as we know, fitness is only one half of the whole—food and nutrition being the other elemental half, and one that matters critically in your mission to run a healthy home. We will start from scratch with regard to nutrition—emptying refrigerators and cupboards of those items that have no role in our master plan of optimal health, and learning how grocery shopping with kids can be a fantastic opportunity to educate them about their food. We will share how to make the entire life cycle of food a collective experience, with tips like family trips to farms, where you can pick your own produce as a team, and the always gratifying act of planting and caring for an herb garden at home together. Finally, we will look at healthy, quick, kid-friendly recipes that are easy on Mom and Dad and still bring on the smiles.

The bottom line is this: Kids learn from example—it's not "do as I say" but instead "do as I do." If they see families who are healthy, active, joyful, and generally well, they will know that healthy lifestyles are a good thing. They will mimic. They will copy. They will imitate. That's why we, more than anything, need to *lead by example*. Plant the seeds of wisdom now, and your family will flourish into a group of strong, vibrant, powerful individuals—all fueled by the same desire to live well.

So we invite you to embrace our mantra—healthier families equal stronger individuals—and let the games and the gourmandizing begin.

Getting Organized

A Call to Rise

Mission: Optimal Group Wellness

If you are a mother or a father, we invite you to—no, we *insist* that you—redefine exactly what that means, starting right now. We invite you to look in the mirror, and in that reflection, see beyond your outdated, preconceived, and preconditioned sense of what it means to be a parent. Instead, we dare you to see a teacher. See a coach. See a chef. See a nutritionist. See a hype man. See a buddy. See an instigator. See a motivator. See a confidante; a mentor; a champion; a challenger. See a partner. See a role model. See a fighter. See a winner. See *and feel* all of these new dimensions as part of your newly revamped role as a mother or a father. Give yourself the eye of the tiger, and commit to a serious-business, you-mean-it paradigm shift in your household, all fueled by the desire to make your family healthier and happier. As parents, we are at the helm of some very special entities—our precious families—and, as the designated adults in the mix, it is our job not only to take care of our children and provide the basics that we already know about, like food and shelter, but also to feed them tirelessly with wisdom and love. But let's leave all the sweet stuff aside for a second and get down to business.

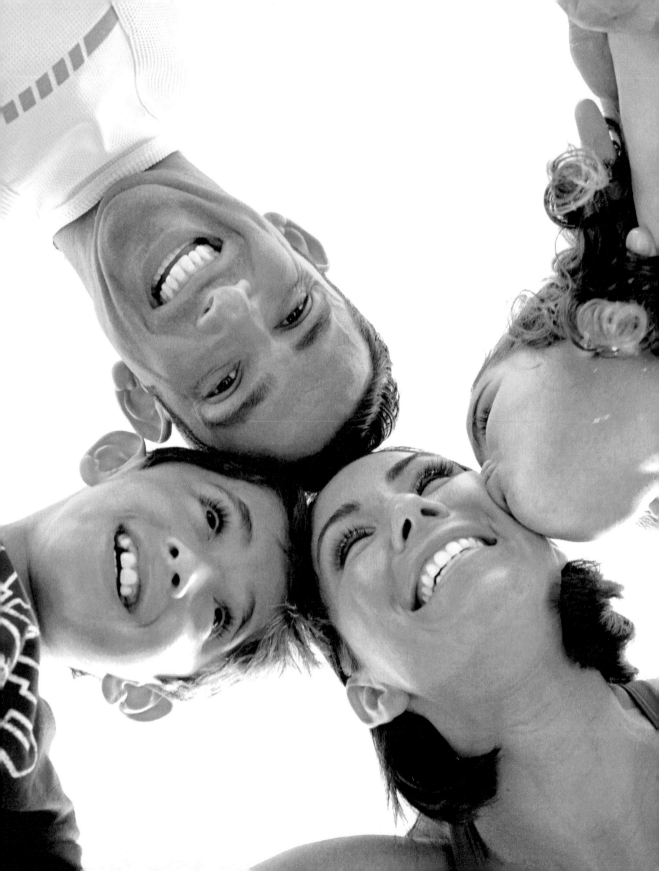

We believe that in order to start something, you have to be willing to *ignite* something, which is exactly how we suggest you begin. Sometimes it takes a little passion and creativity to make a point. For example: make it a point to call an all-important family meeting, with a serious look in your eye but a playful smirk on your face, a vibe that signals to your kids that something interesting and fun is about to happen. Take it seriously by showing up with a clipboard and a whistle. Play the part of team leader with real gusto, and zone them in—wake everybody up, shake them from their laze and haze, because from this moment forward, through this *call to rise,* you declare to the members of your family that happiness will be defined in the context of group wellness and health.

Explain to your children, with a tone and attitude that you know will engage their interest and curiosity, about the fundamental merits of true wellness, and what it could mean to live an exceptionally strong life of excellent health. Make it clear to everyone that this is the dawn of a new era for the family, one based on fortitude and wisdom—as individuals and, what's more important, as a family. Get everyone excited about the prospect of partaking in thrilling activities and games, interesting new foods and recipes, day trips and seasonal excursions.

Tell them that changes are coming, the kind that will make their lives immeasurably better and endlessly more fun. Obviously, kids will have a hard time understanding the importance of longevity and wellness, given their inborn sense of invincibility—so remember to keep it fun, playful, and in the spirit of good times a-comin'.

Growing up, we did not live in the technologically developed game-playing society that our children inhabit today, each with their own laptop, PDA, Game Boy, and all other varieties of simulated recreation; we did not have virtual video games, cell phones, pagers, or computers that could download whatever our little hearts desired at the drop of a hat. All we had were our God-given imaginations, which is exactly what we were forced to tap into if we wanted to have a good time. *And we had a great time*. It was the old-school classics, like tag, hide-and-seek, monkey in the middle, and tug-of-war that, despite being basic and stripped-down, engaged our spirits and kept our little bodies strong. Most significantly, these were the very games that created some of our fondest childhood memories.

Maybe tell your family a bit about the tragedy of the obesity epidemic in the United States, and how unfortunate the whole thing is, considering that being healthy can actually be fun. Explain to them that a healthy body equals a healthy mind, and convince them that it is possible to have both and at the same time entertain quality family time. Make it known to them that moving forward, the family, as a group, will commit to making these key changes toward health and wellness. The changes will mostly affect food and fitness, but above everything they should reflect a profound change of your collective attitude— one that promotes strength, love, health, and joy. Start to make *healthy* the operative word when making decisions about food or fun, and get everyone excited about the prospect of making a "healthy choice" as often as possible. Perhaps even tell them that the person who wins in the end is the one who made the most healthy choices. Lure them in to this concept and have fun with it. Explain to your family that this meeting marks the start of your very own Fit Home Team Challenge—and get everyone revved up about the pleasure and games that are about to begin. Get your spouse involved. Do anything you have to do, but do whatever it takes to *ignite something*.

Congratulations. You have gotten everyone excited, the mojos are rising, people are happy, and the momentum is yours. Time to lay down some ground rules. These rules, as you will explain, will serve as the basic code of behavior (and even attitude) that everyone will agree to honor. This has to be emphasized, so do whatever you have to do to make it clear. Insist that everyone (yourselves included) promise to keep all of these rules as often as possible. Write up a contract. Make it official. Make it matter. And most important, make it *FUN*.

THE S (AS IN SUCCESS!) LIST

Safety

Safety first. It's a cliché because it's true. Safety does come first, and that is exactly why we're starting here. For every activity, every game, every sport, *everything* that we discuss in this book, safety should always be the number-one measure that we check against and the first thing we think about before we do anything. Safety includes the obvious, like having the proper gear and equipment for activities such as soccer and in-line skating, and sunscreen at the beach; as well as other, less obvious, practices, such as knowing some first aid. You might suggest that the family take a CPR class to pick up some basics. Instill in your kids the concept that any sense of fun has to begin by respecting safety, and make them promise that they will always aim to be conscious of it. That said, as the adult(s) in charge, you too should familiarize yourself with any relevant safety measures that correspond to games or activities that you will lead the family in.

Sunshine

Rule number two: When the sun is out, we should be too. Say good-bye to lazy afternoons in front of the television or playing video games on a perfectly crisp and gorgeous blue day. The sun should be your *reason* to be outside, and your family should make it its mission to live in its warmth as often as possible. Granted, sunscreen is *always* a must, and one quick internet search on the dangers on sunburns should answer any questions you may have about this, but assuming you are diligent in your sunscreen application (for your kids and yourselves!), you should relish in the positivity (and vitamin D) that come directly from the rays of the sun.

Sleep

Early to bed, early to rise, makes a man healthy, happy, and wise. We believe it, and we try to keep to that schedule as often as possible. Granted, we're not tyrants about it, and there are plenty of weekends when we all stay up late watching movies, laughing, and having a grand old time. However, as a basic premise, we like to teach our kids that sleep, like nutrition and exercise, is one of the best-kept little secrets for optimal health. Proper sleep leads to energized days, allowing the body to rest, recover, and rev itself up for what is to come.

Stretching

This one falls under the golden rule of safety and therefore is a necessity every single time anyone in the family is going to partake in any physical activity, whether as a group or on their own. The beauty of stretching is that anyone can do it, at any age, and it is always healthy and advisable. Getting your children in the habit of stretching when they engage in physical activity not only helps increase range of motion but also warms the muscles up for the work ahead, stimulating better circulation, which in turn leads to better coordination. Postexercise stretching also helps to decrease muscle soreness and ensure that the muscles and tendons work well. The more conditioned the muscles and tendons are, the better they can handle the rigors of sport and exercise, and the less likely that they'll become injured. So why not start them young? (See page 125 in the fitness section for suggestions on good stretches for kids.)

Sharing

This is another biggie, especially when you are dealing with younger children who are still in the throes of ethical development or siblings who like to have a go at one another when it comes to "their stuff." All very normal, we know. But since we are going to be working with all kinds of sporting equipment and other activity props, it is crucial to state right from the start that sharing is the only way things are going to run smoothly. Make it part of the "groupthink" ideology, and establish right up front that sharing should and will underscore any activity that requires "things." Make it a "what's-mine-is-yours"

atmosphere, and ensure that the little ones especially understand the importance of this rule.

Storing

Teaching your children about order and tidiness isn't just for
your Fit Home Team Challenge—it will be something invaluable
that hopefully they will carry on for the rest of their lives. Stor-
ing, putting things away, organizing, cleaning up—these are all
activities where everyone can chip in, be it in the backyard, the
kitchen, their bedrooms, or the den. Make the cleanup all part
of the challenge, and make everyone accountable for something each time. This helps to foster a sense of collaboration
and unity—not to mention the whole point of keeping a neat,
mess-free home, which is to impart a sense of calm and secu-
rity, and to avoid wasting time looking for things.

Sportsmanship

We believe that being a good sport is one of the secrets to
being a good person, and this code of ethics is part and parcel
of every single game we play as a family. Sports have taught us
both so much about life—they taught us how to win and they
taught us how to lose, mostly because they showed us how one
is *treated* when one is a winner, and how it *feels* to be a winner
or loser. Both are valid experiences by virtue of the extraor-
dinarily useful lessons that they carry. Kids' egos are delicate
little things, which is why it is great to get them into the idea
of letting go of theirs from an early age—which is exactly what

good sportsmanship is all about. Granted, the whole concept of the Fit Home Team Challenge is meant to stir your family's "winner" itch; but just as significant will be everyone's ability to accept the reality of losing, and the understanding that the point is as much to enjoy as it is to be the undisputed champ. Teach your kids to be gracious, not to brag if they excel, to always shake hands, to really grasp the notion that it is *all in good fun*. Maybe explain to them that in sports, team captains are usually selected not on the basis of how good they are but rather in terms of their ability to be a solid team player.

Supplements

Taking the right vitamins and minerals is just as important as eating the right kinds of foods, so part of the new Fit Home initiative will be to get your crew into the mind-set of supplementing their nutrition with all the right stuff. If that means you have to feed your kids vitamins in the shapes of cartoon characters, so be it—but do what you must to get everyone their daily dose of the needed nutrients. A good multivitamin is ideal, and it can easily become part of everyone's morning routine. In addition, you should address any special needs, such as iron deficiencies and so on, of individual family members.

Sitting Together to Eat

We live in a society where teenagers throw Pop-Tarts into the toaster, call it dinner, and run out the door, while parents, in their effort to "be cool," casually allow the television to be on during meals. In Latino homes, sitting together for dinner was always paramount, and when we were kids, this was one of those holy grails that you just didn't argue with. Today we are endlessly grateful for the strictness imparted to us regarding family meals, and thankfully, we matured into adults who actually think the really "cool" thing to do is enforce this rule with our own kids. Mealtimes are some of the few shared moments, when all the members of the family can take a break from their own agendas—work, school, or any other such obligations—and simply enjoy one another's company, sharing in the miracle and joy that is *family*. Teaching your kids not to take these precious moments for granted, as we see it, fortifies them with the wisdom that true kinship is the most beautiful thing out there.

WRITE ON

When we write things down, we essentially account for them—so keeping track of the family's progress, literally, will be key on the path toward fitness and health. You will see that taking notes is a surprisingly effective way to stay connected with your progress, as it asks you to chronicle your behavior, which forces you, as a group, to see where the bad habits and mistakes occur. See the chart at the back of the book on page 200, which you can pin up on your fridge and use as a reference against your shopping list next time you are in the store—a great way to keep the menus varied and dynamic. Every Sunday, sit down with your family and check your progress. This is also a great opportunity to catch up on other events in your kids' lives and to work together as a team toward a healthy family lifestyle.

Taking Stock, and the Art of Always Being Ready

Have you ever noticed how sometimes the hardest part about anything is actually to be prepared, and how, when you actually *are* prepared, the "hard part" seems to be over and done with? Consider the following example: you want more than anything to whip up the most savory chicken soup, replete with all varieties of veggies, herbs, and fixings—however, you wish desperately that someone would just chop up all of your ingredients, line them up in perfect little bowls, like they do on the cooking shows on TV, and even wash your knives right up front, before the soup begins to simmer. Why do you wish these things? We are sure it is not because you are lazy, untalented, or stupid. *It's because you want to be ready.* Because in life, as in the kitchen, everything is so much smoother and less frenetic when you actually take the time to prepare.

Think of being ready as "the art of the head start," poising you for whatever it is you are about to face—which, in our case, will mean a couple things: first, in fitness we have to ensure that all of our sporting goods, props, toys, and safety gear are in place; second, in the kitchen we have to take stock of all of the relevant necessities that we may require, from ingredients to tools. If we are ready on both of these critical fronts, we are ready to be collectively healthy.

Let us be clear: being ready is more than just for the sake of being ready, and trust us when we tell you that our agenda in this discussion on preparedness is not because we want you to be unshakably nerdy or anal-retentive about how you run your show. Instead, we bring up this concept for one simple reason, which is that *being ready is a natural motivator.* Think about it; it's really very simple. If you have the right kinds of food in your fridge, you will be more inclined to eat right; so too, if you have the right kind of equipment in your house, in your backyard, by the pool, and so on, you are more likely to engage in those activities and games that call on such gear. It's the basic law of cause and effect at play, in the context of at-home decision making, and with your family as the point of it all.

Be resourceful. Take a good long look around your house and reinvent it somehow as a gym. Where is there an open area for stretching? Where can you keep some balance/medicine balls around? Which chairs can we use for arm exercises? Are there any sharp edges we should be aware of? Take stock, and be creative about your space and its own resources. If you have a swimming pool, for example, that is a major plus, and know that from this moment on, you are really going to maximize its use (weather permitting, of course). So now that you under-stand how being ready is the root of organization and motiva-tion, let's take a look at what this really means for you.

If we are indeed committed to embarking on a full-on Fit Home Team Challenge, the first order of business will be to stock up on the gear. "The gear" refers to all of the perennial must-haves—in the kitchen and beyond—that should be readily accessible in your household to actualize your campaign of fitness and health. Remember to keep everything organized and labeled, so that your house does not turn into a storage facility, and maybe assign each child (if applicable) different responsibilities for keeping everything clean and stored. You don't have to be a drill sergeant, but again, explain that tidiness is also part of the healthy agenda that we're all trying to get behind.

Since we know that our family health and wellness program is a two-pronged challenge—one being fitness and the other being nutrition—we also need to make sure that our kitchens are devoid of the toxic stuff and chock-full of all the right elements; this means having at hand not only the right foods and the right ingredients but also the necessary tools that will make every mealtime a piece of cake, so to speak. If it is possible, we recommend the following must-haves for your kitchen. (In the chapter that follows, we will review this list in more detail.)

Kitchen Basics

Juicer

Blender

Chopper or food processor

A good set of knives (for adults' use only!)

A fresh herb garden

Plastic lidded containers, assorted sizes

Ziplock bags and aluminum wrap

Disposable plates, cups, and bowls in fun colors

Fresh fruits and veggies in the fridge, peeled and sliced

Popsicle trays in fun shapes

Toothpicks (kids love things on toothpicks; don't ask us why)

Water cooler with accessible cups nearby

Kids are all about attention span, so if you want to deliver for them, you simply must have your bag of tricks. This can literally be a giant bag that you fill with gear. Kids love variety, and your bag of tricks will vary depending on the season. Your job should always be to aim to entertain. The more you have handy, the more fun everyone can have. It's easy. Your summer bag has a Frisbee, sunscreen, beach ball, clean towels, goggles, paddles and ball, Velcro catch kit . . . you get the picture. The bag ensures your readiness and poises you to engage in these activities. It takes the hassle out of last-minute preparations and frees you up to play on the spot. Think of the following as a starting point hit list, and trust that your kids will get excited when they see the house abundant with such goodies.

The Gear

Various sizes and styles of balls (beach ball, soccer ball, etc.)

Mats for stretching and yoga

Sunscreen

Bikes and bicycle helmets

Jump rope

Timer

Stepper

Frisbee and flying disk

Hula hoop

In-line skates

Athletic clothes, shorts, socks, sneakers, etc.

Knee and elbow safety pads

Boxing gloves (sizes for everyone)

Baseball bat, ball, and glove

Heavy, sturdy rope (for climbing and tug-of-war)

Gardening supplies: hose, watering pitcher, shovels, etc.

Balance and medicine balls

iPod with portable speakers or any other music-playing device that's easy to carry around

Basic first aid kit

You've done the hard part; you've assembled your gear and your tools, and hopefully you've done your best to pep up your home team in the spirit of smart, healthy living. Now you're ready to really get cooking, which is why we now move, quite naturally, to the topic of food.

Food Matters

The New Mood on Food

All the efforts and exertions that we practice during our family campaign of health and wellness certainly matter, as this is the outward, external hard work that keeps the furnace active. But just as critical, and on an entirely different level of importance, is the internal work—rethinking every detail of *what we consume*—because food *is* the fuel that keeps that human furnace burning and alive. As parents we are so caught up in all the potential "dangers" our children face, and we spend our lives trying tirelessly to protect them from absolutely everything—when one of the most basic levels of protection can—no, *must*—begin with what we feed them or even allow them to eat. Let us consider a massive priority readjustment when it comes to food.

What is it about our society that teaches children that candy and junk food are OK? They are so *not* OK. As adults we know, from the zillions of diets out there preaching the adverse effects of sugar on health and weight loss, that we should stay away from sugar at all costs. So why on earth do we feed it to our kids? And we *do* feed it to our kids: it's in their breakfast cereals, in their chocolate milk, in their candy bars, in their ice cream treats, in their fruit juice, and in countless other offenders that sneak

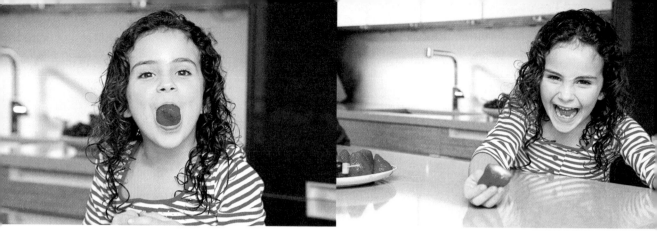

unnecessary sugar into our families. Though we shouldn't be tyrannical in our rage against sugar, the truth is that nature herself makes plenty of it organically, which you know if you have ever tasted the nectar of a ripe summer peach or a sun-ripened mango in the heat of the tropics. There are plenty of "good" sugars, carbs, and fats out there for life to be consistently savory and sweet and simply delectable every single day.

This section aims to help rewrite your family "script" for food, cooking, and eating, and to help shape an entirely new attitude toward what you bring to your kitchen. It is an invitation for you to tap into your inner chef, giving you a moment to shine, by using your skills and savvy to reinvent your kitchen as a source of delicious and nutritious possibilities. For us, the culinary inspiration has always been strong. Having grown up in Puerto Rico and lived in places like Florida, New Orleans, and New York, we have had the good fortune of sampling many varieties of tastes and cuisines. We bring this very inspiration, combined with our knowledge of what is healthy, to our table every day.

We also believe that food is an extraordinary way to educate your children, because every vegetable and every fruit that they will ever eat has a story, such as how it was farmed, when it is in season, how to peel it, and so on. The more you teach your children about where their food comes from, the

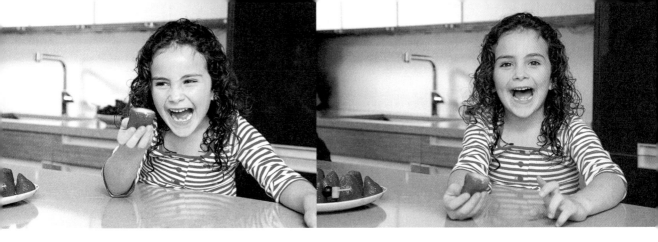

more you help them connect with the earth and also with the art and culture of eating. They won't take their produce for granted when, for example, they are able to grow their own tomatoes or try to keep a basil plant alive. Show them the delight of gardening from an early age and you are essentially teaching them about the beauty of personal gratification and fulfillment. If you think about it, planting and gardening are such primal things—ancient cultures must have taught their young about their merits all along. Why not get your kids into it early in their lives? They will thank you for it later when they are able to grow all their own herbs, and maybe even vegetables.

Here's something else to consider: although we wrote this book as a preventive tool to guide you on your family path of health and wellness, it is likely that some of you are already contending with overweight kids who seem to be on a downward spiral. The challenge of dealing with weight issues during childhood is that you want to slow down the rate of the weight gain without compromising normal growth and development. For this reason, the best thing we can do is to bypass altogether the *need* for childhood weight loss, by exercising the right kinds of choices at home from the moment our children come into the world.

This practice begins with your commitment to getting creative about the recipes you use at home and demands that you keep your radar up as to what will appeal to your kids. Learn the character of your little ones' taste buds and allow your shopping and cooking to be an exploration, with them, of the cuisines of the world—and about the *right* kinds of cuisine. It doesn't have to be fancy: it is as simple as stewing vegetables in coconut milk (which happens to be exceptionally nutritious) and crushing peanuts on top to teach your family about an aspect of Thai cooking. In this way, you can begin to let the world into your kitchen, one meal at a time. You can have global theme nights—Mexican, Italian, Japanese—you get the picture. When you shift your attitude about what you feed to your family and start to have fun with the nourishing possibilities, palates are stimulated and bodies are healthy.

JUNK PURGE

First things first: if there's junk in your house, it's got to go. There are no two ways about it. Throw it out, give it away, do whatever you have to do, but get it out of your kitchen and out of your life. When you purge your cupboards and fridge of the toxic stuff, you essentially clean the slate and make room for healthy business. The junk purge is the first step on the path, and it absolutely *has* to happen. So roll up your sleeves, be strict in your edit, get rid of anything loaded with sugar, and lose as many of your processed foods as possible too. Remember that as your children grow and develop, nutrient-rich foods are the building materials that their brains will require to run properly. The brain needs carbohydrates for energy and pro-

When I went away to college, as athletic and fit as I had always fancied myself, I still managed to put on those dreaded "Freshman Fifteen," which of course was a total outrage to my friends and family when I showed up in Puerto Rico looking rather plump after a year of burgers, pizza, and the like. I tried all varieties of diets and regimens, including not eating. At one point my daily intake consisted of salads and candy bars. It was wrong, and I guess I knew it intuitively. So did my mother, who was a practicing nutritionist. She explained that if I wanted to shed my unwanted pounds, I would have to do it the old-fashioned way: healthy, clean, nutritious eating, lots of water, and exercise. Today, making these choices is so much easier for me, because, along with my husband (who must also eat right not just for the sake of his health but for that of his profession as a serious athlete), we are able to make healthy choices as a team, which not only makes the process easier and more fun but also allows us to show our children the path to proper nutrition.

—*Laura Posada*

teins and healthy fats to build connective pathways between the brain cells. Vitamins, minerals, and other essential nutrients in the right foods help create the neurotransmitters that relay signals between the brain cells.

With this in mind, moving forward, we are going to be thinking in terms of a diet composed of "whole" foods (or foods that are as close to their original state as possible)—moving further away from things full of chemicals and closer to unprocessed things like fruits, vegetables, lean proteins, whole grains, as well as lots of water. Look at the nutrition labels on the backs of your products and really keep an eye out for sugar and excessive or bad fats. As a guiding principle, get rid of high-calorie food that has low nutritional value—commonly known as *junk food*. It is important for us to redefine, in a sense, what we view as junk food, as we are now no longer talking simply about products like fried fast food and potato chips, which are obvious no-nos. Think instead of junk food as a spectrum; the foods with the most nutritional content are those that are fresh, whole, and un-processed; conversely, "junk" constitutes everything made with lots of additives, sugar, unnaturally high fat content and trans fats—the kind of stuff that keeps in your pantries for ages. Think *fresh,* be it protein or vegetables, and start to broaden your understanding of junk food by knowing that the more a food product has been modified, the worse it will be for your body. Make your junk food truly junk by getting rid of it.

According to the U.S. Department of Health and Human Services, many people consume more calories than they re-quire, yet without meeting their basic nutrient needs. With this in mind, now that we're in the process of purging, let's start to focus on choosing food items that are low in calories and high in nutrients—foods that will aid in our kids' normal growth without making them gain unnecessary weight. Other culprits that we should also start to avoid are cholesterol, saturated and trans fats, sugars, and salt, so if you see these villains lurk-ing quietly in your pantry, stand there with both hands on your hips, tell 'em there's a new sheriff in town, and kick them out of the house.

You will see how liberating it feels to see your kitchen

through the new eyes of well-being. If your kids object, as they very likely might when they see their Heath Bar Crunch ice cream bars being shipped off to the garbage, explain to them that sugar comes in many forms, and promise that you will introduce new forms of sweet fixes as part of this new family challenge.

SHOPPING SMART

One of the most freeing concepts for all moms should be that buying groceries is not, and should not, be relegated just to mothers. In fact, the more everyone is involved in the process of selecting and rejecting food items for the home, the more suitable all the meals will be for everyone's unique palate. And, more to the point, the whole endeavor will become a collective effort, giving parents a distinct opportunity to teach while at the store, by showing children through example how to shop the healthy way. You'll see that this basic activity of shopping as a group can naturally help instill awareness and wisdom into the family perspective on food. And it invites *you* to transform what you may once have thought of as a lonely and tedious chore into an opportunity to educate *and* hang out with your family.

In Puerto Rico, where we grew up, though our fathers were very macho in their demeanor, they were never too macho to take us to the grocery store, where they would methodically teach us, in specific detail, how to choose this or that fruit or vegetable. It was not uncommon for our fathers to hold a tomato up to eye level, assessing it as they would a potential bride for a son. They would show us the differences between a good avocado and a great avocado; they would make us smell the ripeness of a perfect grapefruit. They would dig through the apples as if they were searching for gold. They would indulge all of our senses and feed our minds in the process of feeding our bellies. As little kids we were quickly bored by the in-store lectures, but today we are so grateful for those lessons, basic life lessons, which essentially teach about the pursuit of *quality* and which we continue to pass along to our own kids when we go to the store. And it doesn't stop there; you should also teach your kids to compare prices and to not just throw things willy-nilly into the cart without first making sure they are the right things to throw in there. As you educate your children about economizing at the store, they will quickly learn the lesson that buying whole, natural foods, like fruits and vegetables, is actually less expensive than buying canned or processed foods.

Grocery shopping with your kids is not only fun but also *crucial,* when you think about how important it is to educate them about nutrition. And what better way to start that process than by showing them, through example, what the smart choices are right there at the store? If they watch you shop smart, they will quickly start to see the building blocks of proper nutrition and to understand that healthy food comes from healthy ingredients. By getting them involved in the shopping, you are getting them involved in the mind-set.

Start by making lists together at home, and ensure that everyone gets to pick their favorites. Make rules like "Everyone has to pick their three favorite vegetables!" And sure enough, you'll have a wide range of vegetable dishes to work with for the week, handpicked by your kid(s). Total win-win. We really believe it is all about getting kids excited about things.

Growing up in Puerto Rico, the roads were not as paved and polished as they are today, and driving to our grandparents' home in San Sebastian meant a three-hour journey that would seem to last for all eternity for us young ones in the backseat, who would complain of the heat and count down the minutes until the moment of arrival. However, what we did know was that halfway through said journey, we would encounter the magical fruit vendors by the side of the road, their kiosks brimming with pineapple so sweet that it tasted like candy to us, and sugar cane and mangos, whose nectars quenched our thirst like nothing else in the world. The fruit meant we were halfway there, and though the trip was far and the hours felt long, our father would somehow always make an experience of it—and the savoring of these fruits in this context, for some reason, will always linger in my memory.

Along with that delicious memory is the vision of my smiling grandparents in the distance as we arrived at their home, as they waved their arms at us, surrounded by the glory of trees dripping with the most luscious tropical fruits like acerola, avocado, mango, orange, grapefruit, and mamonsillo.

After an entire childhood of these lovely exchanges, today we like to show our own kids that a good piece of fruit at the right time is nothing short of a small slice of heaven.

—*Laura Posada*

Don't just absentmindedly throw things into your cart; instead, show your kids that you take the time to read the nutritional information—*and actually read the nutritional information*. Show them that the whole process, from the store to the kitchen, should be done consciously, taking careful stock of what we put into our bodies and being mindful, always, to savor it all.

And did they sneak in artificial sweeteners that you might have otherwise missed since the sugar content might have read zero? Don't stop there. Did they use partially hydrogenated oils? Was it plain old enriched white flour that contributed to the carb content, or did they substitute or combine that with some good quality whole grains?

Also, how long is that ingredient list? Are there tons of really long words that seem to make no sense? Maybe the item is loaded with binders, fillers, and lots of other chemicals that you really don't want your family eating. So be aware, be alert, and become your own food detective right in the store.

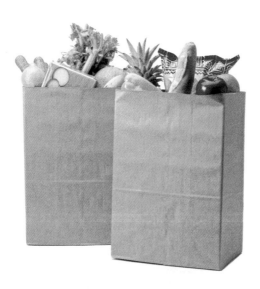

Mission: Nutrition

We know that often the information on some of these labels can be entirely confusing; and for many of us, one quick glance is all we need to "yay or nay" the item, though the truth is that we should all, for our family's sake, be ruthlessly vigilant about which products make it to the checkout line. But since it is unlikely that you will be schooled in the nuances of nutrition overnight, let's go through some of the critical basics, the elemental information (some of which you may already know) that will help make your trips to the store more directed, purposeful, and free of unhealthy choices.

THE FACTS ABOUT FATS

Don't necessarily be put off by the word *fat;* after all, fats supply energy and essential fatty acids, and they play the part of the carriers for the absorption of vitamins A, D, E, and K, which are fat-soluble; as well as carotenoids, which can act as antioxidants. Fats, which exist in foods derived from plants and animals, are the building blocks of membranes and play critical roles in many biological functions. The bottom line is, we need fat, but the key is in the *quality* of the fats you choose.

Nutritional Labels . . . What Gives?

Feeling a little overwhelmed when looking at food labels? Well, don't be. It's really not nearly as confusing as it looks. Each food label is required to show the amount of calories, fat (total, saturated, and trans), cholesterol, sodium, total carbohydrates (broken down into dietary fiber and sugars), protein, and various vitamins and minerals in *one serving* of that particular food. And that is the key right there: the ever-mighty "serving size!" Most people look at these labels and forget to factor in that serving size, and therefore they may think they're consuming a lot fewer calories, fat and carbs than reality dictates. So make sure right off the bat that you look to see what they are referring to as one serving (one cup, one ounce, etc.).

As we continue our discussion of healthy eating, such as good vs. bad fats, the importance of protein, and not overconsuming calories and sodium, you can easily just scroll down the list of nutrients and sum up the food item in seconds. But certainly don't stop there. Probably the best tip we can give you here is to not only scrutinize that food label, watching out for such things as **trans fats, tons of sodium**, and **excessive sugar**, but to continue on and *read the ingredients,* which is a lot like going backstage and seeing what's behind the curtain. Exploring the Ingredient List is just as important, if not more important, in determining whether or not a food will make the cut. This list tells you what type of sweetener they used to sweeten the deal. Was it high fructose corn syrup, or was it simply fruit juice or organic raw sugar?

Because essential fatty acids cannot be made in the body (with the exception of breast milk), you have to ensure your family gets enough of them through the foods they consume.

According to the U.S. Department of Health and Human Services, the recommended total fat intake is:

- 20 to 35 percent of calories for adults

- 30 to 35 percent of calories for children two to three years old

- 25 to 35 percent of calories for children and adolescents

The Fats: Heroes Versus Villains

Fat Types	Fat Sources	Fat Roles
Good Guys *Monounsaturated*	Avocado Olive oil Nuts and seeds Lean protein	Monounsaturated fats can lower cholesterol when they replace saturated fats.
Good Guys *Polyunsaturated*	Salmon Tuna	Does the same as monounsaturated fats and may be even more effective.

(Table continues)

Fat Types	Fat Sources	Fat Roles
Good Guys *Omega-3 (a type of polyunsaturated fat)*	Breast milk Tuna, salmon, mackerel Nuts and flaxseed Soy foods Green leafy vegetables Legumes Walnuts	Omega-3 fats are associated with eye and brain development in utero and during the first six months of a baby's life. As adults, when we consume omega-3 fatty acids, they become absorbed by our different tissues and incorporated mainly into our cell membranes, where they affect the metabolic activities carried out in the cells, sometimes restraining activity, other times facilitating certain functions. For example, these long-chain omega-3 fatty acids are incorporated into the retina of the eye and affect visual function. In the brain, they affect neurodevelopment and function. In the heart, they influence electrical activity to discourage abnormal heart rhythms.
Good Guys *Omega-6 (a type of polyunsaturated fat)*	Vegetable oils like sunflower, peanut, and soy	These protect against heart disease by neutralizing the bad cholesterol.
Bad Guys* *Saturated Fat*	Animal products, such as meat fat; palm oil; coconut oil; high-fat dairy products	Excessive amounts increase bad cholesterol in the body.

Fat Types	Fat Sources	Fat Roles
Worst Guys* *Trans fats* (Hydrogenated Oils)	Commercially made cakes and cookies; shortening, margarine; processed foods, such as chips, energy bars; processed meats and dairy products.	Increases the quantity of bad cholesterol in the body *and* reduces the amount of good cholesterol.

*Get these offenders out of your house during the junk purge!

TAKE IT WITH A (SMALL) GRAIN OF SALT

Salt is one of those things that people only start to get meticulously cautious over if they absolutely must. A middle-aged man with a newly discovered heart condition, for example, will likely curb his sodium intake, as might a bride-to-be trying to quickly drop fifteen pounds before her big day. But often, most of us go straight for the shaker the minute there is a hot plate of eggs, fries, or steak under our noses—and some of the less wary among us take it even further, barely able to eat *anything* without a generous dose of salt. So, of course, our children see these unhealthy habits and mimic, learning—by bad example—to add salt to their own food, with little regard for the unhealthy consequences, which are numerous.

The bottom line about salt is that we should *all* be cautious about our intake, *especially* children, who are still early enough in the game to prevent illness and thwart any damage. Most disconcerting is the recent research showing that young children are eating so much salt that they are suffering from supposedly adult conditions such as high blood pressure, hypertension, and obesity. However, the challenge of monitoring your children's sodium intake can be tricky, mostly because you won't always know what they are being served at their peers' homes, what their lunches are like at school, or how much salt a restaurant uses in the meals your kids order. So here are some basic guidelines to keep the sodium low at least at home:

The Simplest Ways to Cut Down on Salt

- **Check all labels.**

- **Choose low-salt products.**

- **Limit salt use during cooking, and do not leave it on the table while the family eats.**

- **Finally, if you have seriously savory palates at home who can't live without their dash of salt, seek out herbal salt substitutes.**

Don't kid yourself: lowering your family's salt intake is an absolute must. Consider that just about one year ago, the *Journal of the American Heart Association* reported that children who eat less salt end up drinking fewer sugar-sweetened soft drinks and may be at lower risk for obesity, elevated blood pressure, and subsequent heart attack and stroke. It is also important to keep in mind that salt is an inorganic substance that has no real use in the body and in fact can cause the joints to stiffen, besides being associated with hardening of the arteries and kidney disease.

However, you should also remember that sodium, a component of salt, is a very important nutrient for the body. Sodium is one of the body's three major electrolytes (potassium and chloride are the other two). Electrolytes control the fluids going in and out of the body's tissues and cells. Salt (which contains both sodium and chloride) is a major source of electrolytes. When the body becomes dehydrated, it loses fluid and electrolytes. The problem lies in the fact that Americans are consuming way too much salt (sodium) and we are throwing off the balance of other important electrolytes, mainly potassium, which we will read about later.

WHAT'S UP, SUGAR?

This sweetest of substances is one of the most addictive flavors in the world and therefore possibly one of the most dangerous for our children, and certainly ourselves. Sugar is one of those devilish things that can sneak into our sense of craving and desire early in our lives, and for some people it becomes the ultimate challenge to cut back. Even worse, it is widely known that many food producers sneak insulin-spiking sugars into their products to increase the flavor when salt and fat have been reduced.

We would like to offer a rethinking of sugar, one that asks you to consider other ways of getting a sugar fix without having to worry about all of the well-known adverse effects of too much sugar, not the least of which are serious diseases such as diabetes and obesity. We like to believe that sugar tastes the sweetest when it comes directly from the gifts of nature.

According to nutritionists, it is the high-glycemic sugars that you have to really watch out for. These include sucrose, glucose, dextrose, evaporated cane juice, maltodextrin, galactose, corn syrup, dextrin, beet sugar, raw sugar, white sugar, concentrated fruit juice, syrup, sorghum, honey, maple syrup, and high-fructose syrup. Foods like soft drinks, ice cream, pastries, canned fruit, and candy are also loaded with starches that inevitably become high-glycemic sugars.

Ways to Moderate Your Family's Sugar Intake

- Buy unsweetened cereal and add fresh fruit and honey at home.

- Stay away from fruit juices that say "from concentrate" and look instead for "100 percent fruit juice." But don't believe the "100 percent" part; you can assume there is still way too much sugar in there. The best thing to do is to dilute the juice at home. This way you can really minimize the amount of sugar per drink but still get a nice kick of flavor too.

- Don't put ketchup at the table for every meal; in fact, try to get your kids accustomed to eating without it. Believe it or not, there is 1 tablespoon of added sugar in every tablespoon of ketchup.

- If your kids love chocolate, introduce them to dark chocolate and see if they bite . . . the closer chocolate is to raw cacao, the better it is for your health.

- Replace maple syrup, for example, with regular honey or date honey; or use natural agave syrup as a sweetener, which is so much better for you than anything with chemicals in it and tastes perfectly sweet in just about anything.

■ Serve a fresh chopped mango for dessert instead of cake or cookies, and teach your family to appreciate this unique, natural sweetness that comes from perfectly ripe fruit. The trick is to eat the right fruits at the right time, and if you stick to this seasonal cue, you'll never miss out on the sweetness factor.

■ Expose your children to fruits like dates and figs, which taste almost like morsels of caramel and also happen to be high in fiber.

THE WHOLE TRUTH ABOUT WHOLE GRAINS

"Whole grain" means that all three parts of the grain—bran, germ, and endosperm—are present. Whole grains are excellent sources of B vitamins, vitamin E, magnesium, iron, and fiber, as well as valuable antioxidants that come from the bran and the germ of the grain.

Research has shown that eating whole grains can reduce the risk of certain types of cancers as well as heart disease and type 2 diabetes, and help with general weight management. Children need two to three servings of whole grains per day, and in general, the more whole grains they consume, the better.

Types of whole grains include (but are not limited to): oatmeal, wild rice, brown rice, barley, whole wheat, bulgur, popcorn, barley, whole rye, millet, quinoa, and amaranth.

An easy way to boost the whole-grain factor in your house is by going brown: instead of serving regular linguine or penne, switch to whole wheat pasta or brown rice pasta, which cook and taste just like traditional pasta and go fabulously with all varieties of sauces and toppings. Replace white rice with brown rice, which you can jazz up with raisins, herbs, nuts, and spices. Likewise, rethink your sandwich making, and use whole grain bread instead of standard white bread. White bread is the enemy, people.

LEAN MEAN PROTEIN MACHINE

We cannot say enough about the benefits of eating lean protein—they include sustained energy, mental focus, and muscle and tissue repair. Every cell in the body is composed of protein, which means protein is a critical building block for our proper growth and development. It is not only important to consume enough protein but also to make sure that it is the *right kind of protein*. These proteins include: lean meats, fish, poultry, cheese, milk, soy milk, eggs, peanut butter, beans, tofu, lentils, nuts, seeds, whole grains, and yogurt. How strict you want to get with your protein options can vary; some might consider easing up on red meat consumption by switching to turkey and chicken burgers. Others might start using turkey bacon and chicken sausage instead of pork. You can also try buffalo, a wild-game choice that tastes similar to beef but has better-quality fats. There are other modifications you can make, such as making a bolognese sauce using ground soy protein, and perhaps teaching your kids that white-meat chicken is healthier than dark meat. The main idea is to keep your proteins lean, low in fat and salt, and of good quality. Best is organic (animals grazed on grains or grasses without pesticides) and hormone free. When it comes to protein, whether it is meat or dairy products, quality is key.

Kid-Friendly Protein Ideas

Peanut butter and jelly sandwich on whole wheat bread

Macaroni and cheese with whole wheat or brown rice macaroni

Grilled cheese sandwich using whole wheat bread and low-fat cheese

Tuna fish sandwich on whole wheat bread

Turkey or chicken burger with low-fat cheese and whole wheat bun

Salmon burgers with avocado on whole wheat bun

Cheese pizza on whole wheat crust and low-fat cheese

Eggs with turkey bacon and chicken sausages

Scrambled eggs with low-fat cheese

Whole-grain hot cereal with honey, nuts, and sliced bananas

String cheese or yogurt for snacks between meals

Whole-grain pancakes with maple syrup, bananas, and almonds

Rotisserie chicken with sweet potato French fries

Spiced lentils with brown rice and yogurt

Chicken or fish tacos, burritos, fajitas, or just about anything Mexican-inspired, using whole wheat tortillas and low-fat cheese

Sushi with salmon and mackerel

Spaghetti and meatballs, using lean ground beef and whole wheat pasta

THE DISH ON FISH

Lately there has been much concern over the dangerously high levels of mercury found in a lot of the fish that we consume. Fish such as shark, swordfish, king mackerel, and tilefish have excessively high levels of mercury and should pretty much be off the menu for pregnant women, nursing moms, or children.

The best thing you can do is to check local advisories to determine the safety of fish caught in your area. There is plenty of online information as well, websites such as epa.gov/fishad visories/kids and ewg.org, which teach kids and parents about which fish are high in contaminants. If you're still unsure, limit fish to one portion a week. You can eat up to 12 ounces—two average meals—per week of fish that are lower in mercury, such as shrimp, canned light tuna, salmon, pollock, and catfish. However, albacore tuna should be limited to one serving a week because these older fish can be higher in mercury than the young tuna. Remember that when eating fish in general, children should be served smaller portions than adults.

THE A LIST: VITAMIN A

Vitamin A is key for healthy vision, as it helps the eyes adjust from light to dark conditions (and vice versa). It also promotes tissue and cell growth and helps the immune system fight infections. Although vitamin A is found only in foods of animal origin, some fruits and vegetables contain compounds called carotenoids, which can be converted into vitamin A by the body. Foods that contain vitamin A:

Eggs

Carrots

Sweet potatoes

C TO IT: VITAMIN C

Vitamin C is a powerful antioxidant that promotes healthy blood vessels and gums, helps heal cuts, and fights infections. It can also shorten the duration and intensity of colds. Foods that contain vitamin C:

Oranges and other citrus fruits

Red peppers

Strawberries

Broccoli

Papaya

CASH IN ON CALCIUM

Recent research on nutrition from the American Academy of Pediatrics reports an increasing number of children suffering from an inadequate calcium intake, which could affect proper bone growth and density. Our window of time for proper absorption of calcium into our bones is limited, so it is crucial that we get our kids to consume enough of it while they are young. To help facilitate the absorption of calcium into our bones are vitamin D—from fish oil, egg yolks, D-fortified foods, and sun exposure—and magnesium, from foods such as green leafy vegetables, potatoes, nuts, seeds, whole grains, avocado, peanut butter, and prune juice. The recommended allowances of calcium for children:

1 to 3 years: 500 mg

4 to 8 years: 800 mg

9 to 18 years: 1,300 mg

Starting at age nine, your child needs the highest daily requirement of calcium, 1,300 mg. Three cups of milk a day provides 900 mg. To reach 1,300 mg, consider adding other calcium-rich foods to their diet including food such as:

Dairy products like cheese and yogurt

Eggs

Green leafy vegetables such as kale, spinach, bok choy, and broccoli

Fortified (low-sugar) juices

Fortified (low-sugar) cereals and whole grain breads

Soybeans

Tofu with added calcium sulfate

Frozen yogurt

Almonds

P IS FOR POTASSIUM

Potassium is an essential nutritional mineral and an electrolyte that has the power to build muscle, regulate the heartbeat, and prevent high blood pressure. This key mineral sends oxygen to the brain, which is necessary for muscle contraction. Potassium also helps reduce joint pain, among many other health benefits, and sadly, most of us do not consume the standard daily dose of it that our bodies really need. However, there are some very simple and delicious ways to make sure your potassium levels are met. They include:

Eating chicken and salmon

Snacking on almonds

Eating beans, such as white beans and lima beans

Eating fruits like bananas, cantaloupe, oranges, and avocados

Eating leafy greens like spinach

Eating potatoes and sweet potatoes with the skin on

Eating low-fat dairy products

The recommended dietary intake of potassium ranges from 500 mg to 700 mg per day for infants between 6 and 12 months. Potassium intake for children aged 1 year, and from 2 to 5 years, are around 1,000 mg per day and 1,400 mg per day respectively. Children above 10 years require 1,600 mg of potassium each day. In adults, including pregnant women, potassium depletion can be avoided through the recommended dietary intake of 2,000 mg of potassium per day.

FAMILY FIBER

There is a lot of talk about fiber in diets for grown-ups, but it is perhaps one of the most underestimated and forgotten nutrients when it comes to your kids. Fiber, which we get from eating unrefined carbohydrates such as fresh fruits and beans, helps the digestive process along and also helps prevent against certain types of cancer and constipation. It is also known to prevent diabetes and heart disease, so make sure you add fiber to your list of key nutrients that make it into your family's regimen.

Excellent Sources of Fiber

Whole-grain breads and cereals

Apples

Oranges

Bananas

Berries

Prunes

Pears

Green peas

Legumes (dried beans, split peas, lentils, etc.)

Artichokes

Almonds

Quick Tips to Up the Fiber at Home

Have oatmeal at least twice a week, and sprinkle a little oat bran on top.

Add oat bran to your kids' favorite cereals.

Make whole-grain pancakes with sliced apples, dates, and figs.

Make whole-grain waffles topped with bananas and date honey.

Serve brown or wild rice with beans.

Add whole-grain barley to soups.

Serve slices of apples with peanut butter.

Make fruit salads with pears, apples, bananas, oranges, and berries, and add almonds for a fiber-packed crunch.

Top ice cream, frozen yogurt, or regular yogurt with whole-grain cereal, berries, or almonds for added nutrition and crunch.

IRON MAN

Iron has the crucial role of making hemoglobin, the oxygen-carrying component of red blood cells, which circulate throughout the body, delivering oxygen to all its cells. Without adequate iron, the body cannot make enough red blood cells, and tissues and organs won't get the oxygen they require. Kids require different amounts of iron at various ages and stages. Here are some basic guidelines:

- Breast-fed babies tend to get enough iron from their mothers until 4 to 6 months of age, when iron-fortified cereal is usually introduced.

- Infants at 7 to 12 months need 11 mg of iron a day. Babies younger than 1 year should be given iron-fortified cereal in addition to breast milk or an infant formula supplemented with iron.

- Kids between 1 and 12 years old need 7–10 mg of iron each day.

- Adolescent boys should be getting 11 mg of iron a day and adolescent girls should be getting 15 mg. (This is a time of rapid growth, and teen girls need additional iron to replace what they lose each month when they begin menstruating.)

- Young athletes or active kids who regularly engage in intense exercise tend to lose more iron and may require extra iron in their diets.

Foods That Contain Iron

Enriched grains

Dried beans and peas

Dried fruits

Leafy green vegetables

Iron-fortified breakfast cereals

Dark poultry

Red meat

Tuna

Salmon

Eggs

Tofu

POWER UP: ANTIOXIDANT SUPERFOODS

Antioxidants are the disease-fighting compounds that exist naturally in foods to help our bodies stay strong and healthy. As the body uses oxygen, there are by-products known as "free radicals" that can cause damage to cells. Antioxidants repair these free radicals and are associated with a decreased risk of many chronic diseases. Some examples of antioxidants include beta-carotene; vitamins A, C, and E; lutein; lycopene; and quercetin. If we're smart and take advantage of them by eating the right kinds of foods, known as superfoods, we can increase our immunity and foster optimal cell health through our systems.

Key Superfoods

Apples (e.g., Gala, Granny Smith, Red Delicious)

Apricots

Artichokes

Asparagus

Black beans

Blueberries

Broccoli

Brussels sprouts

Cabbage

Cacao (raw)

Carrots

Cherries

Cranberries

Eggplant

Garlic

Grapefruit

Kale

Kidney beans (red beans)

Kiwi

Lemons

Orange

Peppers

Pineapple

Pinto beans

Plums

Pomegranate

Prunes

Raspberries

Red grapes

Russet potatoes

Soy

Spinach

Sunflower seeds

Sweet pecans

Sweet potatoes

Tomatoes

Walnuts

Whole grains

DRINKING PROBLEMS

One of the most important issues in a family's diet, and often overlooked, is not so much what to eat but what to drink. It is high time to get on the beverage patrol and start realizing that the fluids we take in have benefits and disadvantages too—and that we should be as conscious of them as we are of the food we eat. Start getting everyone into the idea of drinking water, and *choosing* water whenever there are many beverage options to choose from. Of course, there will be other beverages they will consume; but even with those, you can begin to be more watchful. For example:

■ **Drink organic, hormone-free milk. You might consider buying whole milk of this variety and simply lessening your portion sizes, as milk's available calcium is cut in half through the process of pasteurization. Low-fat milk makes calcium unabsorbable because fat is an essential part of the transportation and absorption of calcium.**

■ **Buy only sugar-free juices, or better yet, drink fresh-squeezed juices for optimal nutrition.**

■ **Do not buy any soda.**

■ **If your kids are hell-bent on a soft drink, consider offering them soda water with a bit of fruit juice in it.**

■ **Encourage water drinking throughout the day.**

■ **Sweeten iced tea with honey or agave syrup and use mint leaves to add even more natural flavor.**

- Serve beverage treats like almond or oat milk with sliced bananas.

- Start squeezing fresh lemon juice into your family's water, as lemons are packed with essential vitamins and nutrients, and the acid in lemons is known to help keep the intestinal tract clean.

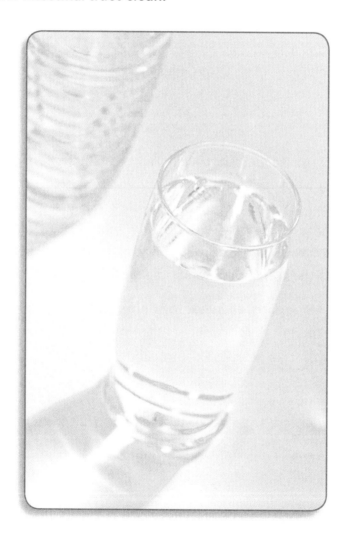

From the Field to the Plate

We will never forget the day in Florida when our son, Jorge Luis, showed up at the front door holding a bunch of lemons freshly fallen from the tree. He held them in the T-shirt he was wearing, folding the front part upward in the shape of a little satchel. He stood there so proudly with his lemons, proud of the fact that they fell off our tree and that he had laboriously picked each one up with his very own hands to make one of his favorite things on the planet: strawberry lemonade. This frosty summer treat takes on a whole new dimension in our house, because our kids love the process of picking the lemons as much as they adore the sweet taste of our delicious drink.

As we see it, the genuine experience of eating well stems from the basic premise of honoring the seasons. What does this mean? It simply means that you should always aim to eat what is in season, which naturally ensures that you are consistently eating fresh; which, in turn, guarantees that everyone has the highest-quality experience of eating produce—and *produce* is exactly what you should be thinking about.

In our family, apple and pumpkin picking are standards every autumn, and strawberry picking is a highlight every

Seasonal Eating 101

Spring produce includes: Artichokes, avocados, asparagus, carrots, fava beans, collard greens, mustard greens, morel mushrooms, mangoes, new potatoes, pineapple, spinach, strawberries, rhubarb, and sugar snap/snowpeas.

Summer produce includes: Beets, blackberries, blueberries, broccoli, cherries, corn, cucumber, eggplant, green beans, nectarines, peaches, plums, raspberries, summer squash, tomatoes, watermelon, and zucchini.

Fall produce includes: Apples, acorn squash, butternut squash, cauliflower, figs, grapes, mushrooms, parsnips, pears, pomegranate, pumpkin, sweet potatoes, and Swiss chard.

Winter produce includes: Chestnuts, grapefruit, kale, leeks, lemons, oranges, radishes, tangerines, and turnips.

spring at a yearly festival in Florida. For us, there is nothing quite like getting our hands dirty with the soil of the earth as we harvest the fruits and vegetables we will be enjoying together at home. Somehow, everything always tastes better to kids when they are involved in the process.

Besides the joys of harvesting, you will be doing your family wonders the moment your menus begin to include more fruits and vegetables. We are pretty sure we don't really have to tell you why. Teach your kids that biting into a perfectly ripe strawberry or lychee can be like eating the sweetest candy treat they have ever tasted.

One of the best ways to amp up the vegetable vibe is to plan family trips for things like fruit picking, or even a day at a farm, where they can learn hands-on from farmers about a specific vegetable; they learn that way so much about how food works. When children have the opportunity to witness firsthand the miraculous cycle of a harvest, they begin to internalize the role it can play in their own lives. They learn about the process of agriculture, and this very knowledge has the power to imbue them with an appreciation for foods that come from the earth, thereby enriching not only their minds but also their diets.

Personal gardening is another way to get people excited. The simple activities of mowing the lawn, picking weeds, or raking up leaves can begin to forge a connection between your family and its environment. All you need is a small wheelbarrow, water bucket, shovel, rake, and gloves, and you are ready to grow. You can take it even further by getting each child to choose an herb of their choice—basil, rosemary, and sage grow well—and allocate an area for the family herb garden, where a little patch of green life can sprout into a lesson for the family on the pleasure and satisfaction of gardening and cooking with one's own herbs. Planting seeds is also known to attract ladybugs and butterflies, which are always delightful little creatures to have around.

You can also make it a point to start visiting your local botanical gardens to get inspiration and to see the flora in its full glory. If your kids really seem to have little green thumbs but you live in an urban area, you might consider joining a community garden where you can volunteer as a group to tend to the communal plot.

Just remember always to keep safety in mind, especially when it comes to gardening. Young children should certainly not handle sharp tools and should be kept far away from any chemicals and insecticides.

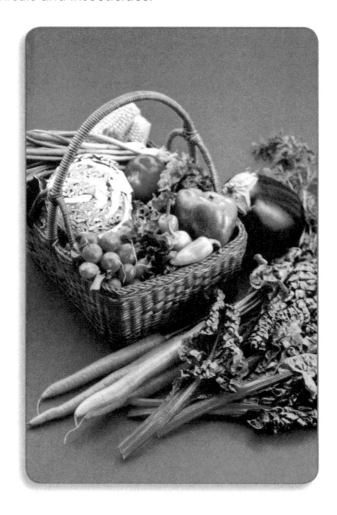

Healthy Craftiness

The Art of Tricking Kids into Wellness

We've been talking about the merits of healthy eating as if children were people who are easily convinced. Raise your hands if your own kids hate fruits and vegetables. It is no secret that most children do not fancy those foods that happen to be the most nutritious. Also, it is important to keep in mind that children's appetites are affected by their growth cycles, and for that reason they have different taste preferences than adults do. We have all heard the term *fussy eater,* which means a child is finicky about what he or she eats. From the age of one to five, it is not uncommon for kids to show erratic appetites, and for a child in the formative years, life is too downright exciting to stop for food.

The good news is that there are all kinds of ways to sneak the good stuff into your kids' diets, clever little culinary schemes that ensure nutrition *and* satisfaction. Your kids will never know what hit them. . . .

Here is our list of clever little things you can do to give your meals an extra kick of nutrients.

SNEAKY TIPS

1. Add fresh blueberries, which are chock-full of antioxidants, to a hot bowl of oatmeal or a bowl of cereal.

2. Roast up some sweet potato fries, which are fun and colorful, and you can season them for an extra kick. Best of all, sweet potatoes are an excellent source of vitamin A.

3. Drizzle honey on fresh fruit, such as sliced apples, strawberries, or pears, and stick toothpicks in them for a quick sweet treat.

4. Make fun-shaped ice pops using freshly squeezed orange juice or other fresh (low-sugar or unsweetened) fruit juices.

5. In general, smoothies are excellent opportunities to sneak in all kinds of nutrients and vitamins—so milk it! There are endless options for yummy smoothies, like raw cacao with vanilla yogurt and honey for a healthy chocolate milk shake, or bananas with low-fat milk, crushed ice, almonds, and dates for a sweet treat we like to call "monkey milk" (see recipes on page 90 for more excellent smoothie ideas).

6. Make fun bowls of healthy trail mix, using almonds, soybeans, raisins, goji berries, and other dried fruit. Keep the bowls out so everyone can nibble.

7. Make homemade soups using fresh vegetables, and zest them up with ginger, coconut milk, and all varieties of herbs and spices. You'll be a star if you add whole wheat croutons, as kids are typically fans of a good crunch.

8. Quiche is another excellent camouflage for vegetables and has the added bonus of eggs, which are high in protein. It is a savory option for breakfast, lunch, or dinner—a meal in a slice.

9. Barbecues are fantastic ways to gather the family and enjoy food the purist way: slow-cooked on a grill over an open fire. Grilled chicken, meats, and vegetables like corn, zucchini, peppers, and broccoli always taste great on the grill. Add a few interesting dipping sauces, like humus or salad dressing, and you cannot go wrong.

10. In the spirit of hands-on foods, start thinking about foods like artichokes, which are fun, unconventional, and interactive and can be kicked up with all varieties of dipping sauces. Interactive fruits that you can peel easily and quickly like tangerines and clementines are also great to have around.

11. Just as effective as the interactive fruits is a heaping bowl of fresh fruit salad. Commit to making one every Sunday night, and you'll see that everyone will pick at it throughout the week.

12. Make it colorful. Kids love things that are brightly colored, and wouldn't you know it—the healthiest foods are popping with hue. Fruits and veggies come in all of the shades of the rainbow; so take this opportunity to make gorgeous canvases out of all your family's meals.

13. Seeing is believing. What we mean by this is that the more your kid *sees* something—i.e., sliced apples on the high-chair tray—the more inclined he or she will be to try them one day. So if you have a finicky eater on your hands who does

not want to taste broccoli, for example, dare to put a few broccoli florets on their plate (and everybody else's, as well, of course) every day—and we can pretty much guarantee that one of those days, they will muster the courage to try it. This rule applies to almost everything your kids are not inclined to try.

14. Make healthy foods more fun and playful by cutting sandwiches, for example, into interesting shapes.

15. Try to keep mealtimes happy, social occasions. Don't get too bent out of shape if a glass of juice is knocked over and spills, and try to keep the general atmosphere of meals positive and joyful. This will condition your kids (especially if they are fussy eaters) to get in on the fun.

16. Bake homemade muffins with your kids, and add carrot, zucchini, and pumpkin to the batter. This proves to them, in a sensory language that they can understand, that vegetables can actually taste delicious.

17. Add chopped veggies such as spinach to soup and pasta sauces; and likewise, add chopped tomato, diced celery, or grated carrots to tuna, chicken, and pasta salads.

18. Make pizza with your kids using a thin crust (ideally whole wheat) and low-fat, part-skim mozzarella cheese, and offer toppings such as chopped broccoli, fresh cherry tomatoes, mushrooms, and spinach.

FOOD = FUN

Going back to the issue of "fussy eaters," for some parents it can seem virtually impossible to get their kids to eat at all, much less eat the right things. We like to believe that the secret ingredient to proper nutrition for children has a lot to do with how much *fun* you inject into the mix. Sitting down for a meal is one thing, but what if that meal involved everyone's participation, creativity, and personal taste? Think about an interactive group gathering where each person "builds" his or her own dish, making it hands-on, stimulating, and totally personal. The point is that kids typically love the idea of collaborating, and everything tastes better to them when they were involved in the process, so get them involved, and you remain the conscious curator about what ingredients they get to play with. Here are some of our favorites.

Sushi Rolling Party

Sushi, a food tradition of Japan, has become a culinary mainstay all around the world, and going out for sushi is as popular today as going out for pizza. We encourage you to take the experience one step further by holding your very own family sushi night, replete with kimonos, chopsticks, wooden blocks, and bamboo rolling mats. You can easily find tips on how to roll sushi—in books, DVDs, and online—or you can wing it and get creative. The nice thing about sushi night is that it encourages your family to eat some of the right kinds of proteins and fats, like salmon and avocado, for example. It also allows you to include sea vegetables, which are rich in nutrients, and other veggies like cucumbers, carrots, daikon root, and sprouts; and if you really want to get serious, you can make your sushi rice using brown rice to add a hearty dose of fiber to the meal.

Taco Night

Our kids love taco nights, and we certainly don't blame them. Who doesn't love a taco night? These Mexican-inspired treats are fantastic because you can make them using whole wheat tortillas and low-fat cheese; serve up excellent protein fillings, such as ground turkey or chicken or lean ground beef; and use all kinds of colorful veggies, like lettuce, tomatoes, avocados, corn, onions, and green, yellow, and red peppers. Another fabulous thing about taco night is that it inspires your kids to try everything, and it puts them in control of their own prefer-ences. Remember that variety is the key to exposing your kids to foods; the more the merrier when it comes to a taco spread.

Salad Bar

OK, we admit it, this is a hard one to pull off, because let's face it, typically kids are not the biggest proponents of . . . well, salad. But you can make salads fun by cutting veggies into cute shapes like hearts and stars and serving salad toppings that your family isn't used to, which always keeps things lively. Think of salad bar night as your opportunity to serve four different kinds of lettuce, so you can observe which ones your kids like the most. Be an investigator, so you can learn about the healthy foods they are attracted to. Serve other healthy items like nuts, seeds, and sprouts, which are excellent sources of nonmeat protein. And as far as dressings go, the key is picking the ones that are not loaded with a laundry list of foreign-sounding ingredients, or simply make your own with olive oil and vinegar (raspberry- or pear-infused) or lemon juice, teaching your kids that less is more, and that what they should really be looking to experience are the distinct flavors of the vegetables. Get them excited about the idea of exploring each taste.

Fro-Yo/Sorbet Sundays

How about a Sunday where you turn your kitchen into an ice cream parlor for an afternoon to make sundaes—except *don't serve ice cream*. Instead, opt for low-fat frozen yogurt or sorbet in a variety of everyone's favorite flavors, and offer up healthy toppings, such as crushed almonds, shredded coconut, raisins, goji berries, and date honey. You can also serve raw cacao nibs instead of chocolate chips—they're lower in sugar but still have the kick; and don't forget to lay out fruit for toppings, like sliced bananas, strawberries, and blueberries.

What's In to Eat when You're Out to Eat

We live in a society where families go out for meals at restaurants just as much as, if not more than, they eat at home. Eating out, though endlessly fun, can have negative effects on your family's nutrition because you don't always know how your meals are being prepared and what is going in them, and because we tend to order things on menus that are less healthy than the kinds of foods we would make for ourselves at home. But if you know you are the kind of family that will inevitably eat out at restaurants a lot, there are small changes your family can make to help keep your restaurant experiences both clean and healthy. It is your job as parents to make sure your kids are well informed about healthy choices versus unhealthy ones, so that when a menu is handed to them, they are already poised to make the right selection.

It is important to teach kids about the nature of "indulgence," and the art of balance and moderation when it comes to eating what they like. As much as we want our children to use wisdom and awareness about what they consume, we also want them to *enjoy* their experience of eating and food, and even revel in some of their favorite tastes and flavors. Eating out is a perfect opportunity to practice this balance as a group, so you should take advantage of these moments to teach everyone about the merits of holding back, alongside the joys of treating oneself.

Here are some basic rules that we like to live by when we go out to eat; we talk about them with our kids, so that the joy of dining out is never taken for granted, and the awareness about food is always present. Let's take a look.

Restaurant Rules 101

- Avoid anything fried or breaded.

- Avoid eating too much (or any) bread before the meal; we sometimes even tell the waiter not to bring any to the table, which helps keep temptation at bay. Frankly, if you're about to consume an entire meal, you certainly don't need to fill up on bread, which is usually white bread anyway. Be warned.

- If you're going to order appetizers, try to keep them salads and veggies. The last thing you need is a meal on top of another meal.

- Sharing is caring, and we love to use the sharing rule when we go out to eat. Restaurant portions are often huge, especially for kids, so sharing main courses is a practical (and economical) way to not waste food (and money). It's also a great way to try various things at once.

- Avoid "kiddie menus," which are usually replete with fried foods like chicken fingers and mozzarella sticks. Instead, make it a game with your kids to identify the healthiest options, even if these happen to be on the grown-up menu, and encourage your children to think like adults when it comes to ordering their food.

- Avoid ordering soft drinks, and instead opt for water all around.

- Avoid adding salt to your meal, as this is typically not something restaurant chefs hold back on in the kitchen.

- Encourage your kids to find the lean protein on the menu, and look for the vegetable sides that they might like.

- Avoid ordering dessert, and instead suggest that you all eat some fruit together when you get home—if anyone even has an appetite by then.

STOP! IN THE NAME OF HEALTH:

Portion Control

There is an expression that says the eyes are bigger than the stomach. We often eat with our eyes, serving ourselves more than we can actually fit into our stomachs. Our society celebrates abundance, and we, little pigs that we can tend to be, indulge the bad habit by overestimating our own capacities. To keep this weakness in check, something that we like to practice is the "stop when you are full" rule; meaning, actually pause to feel the sensation of a having a full belly, take a few deep breaths, and honestly ask yourself, Am I full? And if the answer is yes, *stop eating.* Teach your kids to connect with their bodies by encouraging them to develop this healthy awareness, and you will be simultaneously teaching them about the merits of self-control and physical connectedness as well as the adverse effects of gluttony and even greed.

Teach your children that they do not have to eat until their little tummies feel on the brink of exploding. Explain to them that, though many people love to insist, you don't *have to* eat everything on your plate. Portions are usually way larger than one human needs to eat in one sitting, so there is nothing wrong with eating only what you need to feel satiated. Another thing you can teach them is the "twenty-minute rule," which says that you should wait twenty minutes before serving yourself more food, as twenty minutes give the belly a chance to settle in with new food and therefore make it better able to assess if it really wants or needs any more at all.

Here are some basic measurement guidelines, according to the American Academy of Pediatrics. Children 2 to 3 years old should consume no more than 1,000 calories each day; girls 4 to 8 should consume about 1,200 and boys of the same age 1,400. Girls between 9 and 13 should get about 1,600 calories daily and boys 1,800. Girls 14 to 18 should aim for approximately 1,800 and boys should shoot for around 2,200. For adults, men need about 2,700 calories per day, and women require about 2,000 calories per day. These calories should include:

2 to 5 ounces of lean meat or beans

1 to 2 cups of fruit

1 to 3 cups of vegetables

2 to 7 ounces of whole grains

The Basics

Healthy Recipes That

Never Go Wrong

And when we say "never go wrong," we don't just mean that your family will love these recipes; we are also encouraging you to try these at home on the basis of how user-friendly, time-efficient, and straightforward they are—not to mention how healthy they are as menu options for kids and grown-ups alike. We believe that eating right means two things: eating foods that are healthy for our bodies, and savoring every bite to the end. If you scan through the recipes, though they span the entire globe in style, you will note some basic common denominators: lots of lean protein, low fat content, and an emphasis on fresh fruits and vegetables. No big mystery, right?

In Latino families, the kitchen has historically and culturally been a place where people convene and enjoy one another's company. It is a place of intimate bonds, shared lives, and team efforts. Get your family excited about working in the kitchen as a group, and you will gradually expand the possibilities of the group bond. Eating together is crucial, but imagine how much more fun it can all be when you also *cook* together. Granted, you're not going to give a sharp knife or a hot pot to a child, but there are other ways to get them involved. For example, have your kids wash the produce, which is a great way to show them the importance of doing so. Empower them with that kind of responsibility.

What we hope to inspire *you* to do is to get more creative and playful about how you eat as a family, always keeping the golden rule of "sneaking the good stuff" into tasty, provocative recipes that you know will satisfy everyone. When you are making menu selections, zero in on your protein and vegetables, and then find a way to combine them creatively. Think about it: if you were a kid, you wouldn't appreciate a plate of steamed broccoli being shoved under your nose. Instead, think about sautéing those cancer-fighting florets in some garlic and a dash of sesame oil, add a hint of soy sauce, and you've showed your family a little sliver of China. Dare to rethink your own conceptions about what "healthy food" tastes like, and imagine an entirely new culinary landscape, both sophisticated and savvy, but rooted in the basic tenets of eating *right*. Some little things you can do include changing ordinary burger nights into veggie or salmon burger nights with all the vegetable fixings; or having a baked potato bar night, using fresh sweet potato, chopped-up veggies, and low-fat cheese.

Of course, every family is different. If you are a meat-eating family, you might introduce the concept of "vegetarian night" once a week, and gradually move up to two nights. At the very least, try to keep your beef as lean as possible, and even better, organic. If you are a Latino family, like ours, white rice might be the true culprit. Consider switching to brown rice, even for just a few nights a week. Look long and hard at your family's eating habits, and think about where you can make small changes that will make a big difference.

Mind you, these recipes are not meant to make you (or anyone in your family) thin as a rail; they are, instead, designed to be quick and easy and offer you a variety of wholesome foods that taste delicious, yet also make you all healthy, balanced, strong, and thoroughly nourished. Remember, we are not into fad diets but rather a lasting, lifelong formula for solid, consistent health and wellness.

In the interim, as you sort through your own patterns and habits, we offer you a smattering of some of our own tried-and-tested favorites, some easy, breezy meals that can happen anywhere with little effort, lots of flavor, and loads of nutrients. We hope you enjoy, or as we say in Spanish, *Buen provecho*.

Go Green: Salads

We like to think of every single salad as an opportunity—a chance to pack in all kinds of healthy and diverse nutrients into one delicious bowl of flavor and sensation. Dump the notion that salads are bland or boring, and dare to liven yours up with some of our suggestions, which we serve regularly, alone or as an accompaniment to our meals. Get creative, use the ingredients your family loves the most, and remember to use the salad as an opportunity to introduce all kinds of new ingredients to your family. In our house, we have a rule: everyone has to try everything at least once. You don't have to like it, but you have to commit to at least tasting it once.

Avocado Salad

Prep Time: 10 minutes, plus 30 minutes chilling
Serves 2

2 ripe avocados
2 hard-boiled eggs
1/3 cup chopped chives
1 lime
Salt and pepper
Natural organic yellow corn tortilla chips

Peel avocados and cut into small cubes. Place in a small mixing bowl. Cut eggs in half and discard the yolks. Cut the egg whites into small pieces and add to mixing bowl. Stir in the chives. Squeeze lime into mixture and add salt and pepper to taste. Mix together until it becomes a paste and refrigerate. Chill at least 30 minutes and serve with tortilla chips.

Mango-Avocado Salad

Prep Time: 15 minutes
Serves 4

2 ripe Hass avocados, diced
2 ripe mangoes, peeled and diced
$\frac{1}{2}$ cup chopped cilantro
$\frac{1}{4}$ cup chopped red onion
$\frac{1}{4}$ cup freshly squeezed lime juice
Salt and pepper

Carefully fold all ingredients together in a medium bowl, being cautious not to turn it into a mash. You might add the avocados last, so that they keep their shape. Don't worry about their turning black, as the lime juice will keep them preserved. Season to taste with salt and pepper.

Shrimp Salad

Prep Time: 10 minutes, plus 1 hour chilling
Serves 2 to 3

1 pound large cooked shrimp
1 (14-ounce) can roasted red peppers, diced
1 cubanelle pepper, diced
1 bunch fresh basil, chopped
Extra virgin olive oil
White balsamic pear-infused vinegar (this is a very specific ingredient that may be difficult to find—any white balsamic vinegar works just as well)
Salt and pepper

We like to use the large cooked shrimp because they come clean, with the black vein already removed, ready for preparation, and totally user-friendly. Remove the tails from the shrimp and cut them in half lengthwise. Mix the roasted peppers, cubanelle pepper, and basil with the shrimp. Toss with the oil and vinegar and chill 1 hour before serving. Season to taste.

Tuna and Pasta Salad

Prep Time: 20 minutes, plus 1 hour chilling
Serves 4 to 6

12 ounces whole wheat rotini pasta
1 large can premium light tuna in water, drained
1 (4-ounce) jar capers
1 bunch parsley, chopped
1 (8-ounce) jar red pimentos, diced
1 large tomato, diced

¼ cup extra virgin olive oil
Salt and pepper

Boil the pasta according to the package instructions. In the meantime, mix the remaining ingredients together in a large bowl. When the pasta is ready, drain and rinse with cold water. Add to the bowl, mix well, and season to taste with salt and pepper. Chill 1 hour before serving.

Chicken and Spinach Salad

Prep Time: 15 minutes
Serves 2 to 3

2 boneless, skinless, hormone-free chicken breasts
2 tablespoons extra virgin olive oil, plus more for the dressing
Salt and pepper to taste
1 teaspoon dried oregano
1 (6-ounce) bag organic baby spinach
¼ cup sliced honey-roasted almonds
½ cup dried cranberries
1 (4-ounce) package goat cheese, crumbled
Balsamic vinegar

Chop the chicken into small bite-size pieces. In a medium saucepan on medium heat, sauté with olive oil, salt and pepper, and oregano. Let cool slightly. Mix the remaining ingredients in a bowl, toss with the cooled chicken, and serve drizzled with balsamic vinegar and olive oil, or with a dressing of your choice.

Soup's On

Is there anything more perfectly cozy than a steaming bowl of homemade soup? In our house, soup represents ultimate lounging and leisure, kicking back at home, and getting nourished from some of the healthiest ingredients around—fresh herbs and vegetables. We love making soup because it's the kind of thing you can make on the weekend and enjoy all week as leftovers; it's hassle-free, healthy, and always fills you up. So grab your favorite set of mugs, and get ready to get cozy.

Vegetable Soup

Prep Time: 50 minutes
Serves 6

1 small Spanish onion, chopped
2 green bell peppers, seeded and diced
2 cloves garlic, chopped
1 potato, peeled and cubed
1 sweet potato, peeled and cubed
1 pound butternut squash, peeled and cubed
1 (8-ounce) can Spanish-style tomato sauce
1 (1.5-ounce) packet taco seasoning
Salt and pepper

2 cups organic fat-free chicken stock

1/2 cup *recao* (also known as "long coriander" or "wild coriander"; you can find it in most gourmet or Latin American stores)

1/2 cup chopped Canadian bacon

Place all ingredients in a large pot over medium heat and bring to a boil. Reduce the heat and let the mixture simmer for about 30 minutes, or until the vegetables are soft. Transfer contents of pot to blender and blend until smooth. Season to taste with salt and pepper. Transfer contents back to pot, heat for a moment, and serve.

Tomato-Basil Soup

Prep Time: 15 minutes

Serves 4

1 (28-ounce) can crushed organic Roma-style tomatoes

1 (6-ounce) can tomato paste with Italian herbs

1 (8-ounce) tub fat-free cream cheese with chives

1/2 cup chopped basil leaves

1/2 cup white wine

Salt and pepper

In a large pot, whisk all the ingredients together. Bring to a boil, and continue to whisk until the cream cheese has melted. Transfer contents to a blender. Blend everything into a smooth liquid, and transfer back to pot. Season to taste with salt and pepper. Heat for a moment and serve.

Corn and Chicken Soup

Prep Time: 45 minutes

Serves 4

2 boneless, skinless, hormone-free chicken breasts

2 tablespoons extra virgin olive oil

½ cup chopped yellow onion

2 cloves garlic, chopped

1 (15-ounce) can whole-kernel sweet corn

1 (15-ounce) can hominy (the larger white kernel corn, which you can get in most Latin American grocery stores)

½ cup chopped cilantro

3 cups organic chicken stock

Salt and pepper

1 lemon, cut into wedges (optional)

1 avocado (optional)

Hot sauce (optional)

Chop the chicken into small chunks and place in a medium pot over medium high heat with the olive oil, onions, and garlic. Sauté until the onions are golden and the chicken begins to turn golden brown. We like it when the chicken even gets a bit crispy. Add the corn, hominy, cilantro, and chicken stock and bring to a boil. Reduce the heat to low, cover, and simmer for about 30 minutes. Season to taste with salt and pepper. We like to serve this one with lemon wedges, chopped avocado, and hot sauce.

Posada Protein Favorites

Lean protein is at the core of a sound diet, so we like to keep a diverse array of protein recipe options at our fingertips. These are the classics in our house, inspired by things we have eaten and loved, and revised to meet our standard of nutrition. By keeping the recipes diverse, we never get bored, and still always manage to stay healthy.

Teriyaki Chicken
Prep Time: 20 minutes, plus 30 minutes marinating
Serves 6

4 boneless, skinless, hormone-free chicken breasts
½ teaspoon salt
½ teaspoon pepper
½ cup low-sodium teriyaki sauce
1 bag frozen Asian mixed vegetables
Salt and pepper

Chop the chicken into strips, as if you were going to make fajitas. Marinate the chicken with salt, pepper, and teriyaki sauce for at least 30 minutes. Heat a large nonstick sauté pan over high heat and add the chicken and marinade. Cook for 2 to 3 minutes. Reduce the heat to medium and add the vegetables. Cover and cook 15 minutes more, stirring occasionally. The vegetables will cook nicely in the juices of the chicken and absorb the sweet teriyaki flavor. Season to taste and serve immediately.

Acapulco Tilapia

Prep Time: 25 minutes
Serves 4

4 tilapia fillets
Salt and pepper
$\frac{1}{2}$ cup fat-free mayonnaise
1 (1.5-ounce) package taco seasoning
Extra virgin olive oil to taste
$\frac{1}{4}$ cup fresh squeezed lime juice

Preheat oven to 375 degrees F. Place the fillets in an oven-safe baking dish and season to taste with salt and pepper. Rub the fillets with the fat-free mayonnaise. Sprinkle evenly with the taco seasoning, olive oil, and lime juice. Cover with aluminum foil, so the fish does not dry out, and bake for about 20 minutes, until the fish flakes easily with a fork.

Creole Chilean Sea Bass

Prep Time: 40 minutes

Serves 4

4 Chilean sea bass fillets (or other firm, white-meat fish such as mahimahi)

Salt and pepper

1 yellow onion, finely chopped

3 cloves garlic, minced

1 (8-ounce) jar roasted pimentos, chopped

1 green bell pepper, finely chopped

$\frac{1}{2}$ cup white wine

1 (4-ounce) jar capers

$\frac{1}{4}$ cup sliced salad olives (jarred green olives topped with pimento)

1 cup Spanish-style tomato sauce

$\frac{1}{4}$ cup extra virgin olive oil

Preheat oven to 375 degrees F. Place the fillets in an oven-safe dish and season to taste with salt and pepper. Mix the remaining ingredients in a small bowl and pour over the fillets. Cover with aluminum foil so that the fish does not dry out. Bake for 25 to 30 minutes, until the fillets flake easily with a fork. Season to taste and serve.

Healthy Burger

Prep Time: 20 minutes
Serves 4

1 pound antibiotic-free lean ground sirloin
$\frac{1}{2}$ cup liquid egg whites
12 whole wheat crackers, finely crushed
Salt and pepper
2 teaspoons Worcestershire sauce
Whole wheat burger buns

We like to use antibiotic-free, lean ground sirloin. Instead of egg yolks, we use just the egg whites—and instead of using bread crumbs, we use whole wheat crackers.

Mix the ground beef with the egg whites and the crackers, and form into 4 patties. Heat a grill to medium-high and cook to desired doneness, about 4 to 5 minutes per side for medium. Right before placing them on the grill, sprinkle with salt and pepper to taste. Add Worcestershire sauce for a little kick. Serve on whole wheat buns. You can also serve them with all the fixings, like lettuce, tomato, and onion, and if you want a proper burger meal, roast up some sweet potato fries to serve alongside.

Mex-Asian Tacos

Prep Time: 20 minutes

Serves 4

3 boneless, skinless, hormone-free chicken breasts

Salt and pepper

2 teaspoons extra virgin olive oil

1 (1.5-ounce) package taco seasoning

1 small yellow onion, chopped

1 bunch cilantro, chopped; save some for garnish

1/4 cup low-sodium soy sauce

1 package small whole wheat tortillas

2 slices fresh pineapple, cut into chunks, or 1 (8-ounce) can sugar-free pineapple chunks

1 lime

Tabasco mild jalapeno green pepper sauce

Begin by cutting chicken into bite-size cubes. Season with salt and pepper to taste. Add the olive oil to a large sauté pan over medium-high heat. Once it is warm, add the chicken and taco seasoning and allow it to cook for 6–7 minutes. Lower the heat to medium and add the onions, cilantro, and soy sauce. Cover, reduce heat to medium low, and cook until chicken is cooked through and has a nice orange color, about 8 minutes more.

While the chicken is cooking, warm up the tortillas and cut the lime into four wedges. Now you are ready to serve. First, place the tortillas flat on a plate. Then fill them up with chicken, pineapple, and fresh cilantro on top. For the adults, I suggest a squeeze of lime, and a dash of Tabasco for a little more kick. Roll up the tortillas and enjoy.

Pepper and Onion Tenderloin Tips

Prep Time: 25 minutes
Serves 4

2 pounds beef tenderloin
1 red onion, peeled
1 green pepper, halved and seeds removed
¼ cup soy sauce
Salt and pepper

Use as lean a cut of beef as possible. Slice into strips. Cut the onion and the peppers into strips the same size. Add the meat, vegetables, and soy sauce to a large nonstick sauté pan over medium-high heat and sauté until cooked through, depending on how rare everyone likes their meat. Season to taste with salt and pepper.

Scrambled Egg Whites and Veggies

Prep Time: 20 minutes
Serves 2 to 3

Nonstick cooking spray
$1/2$ small yellow onion, chopped
1 small tomato, chopped
4 slices turkey, chopped
$1/4$ green pepper, chopped
2 cups liquid egg whites
Salt and pepper
$1/3$ cup shredded fat-free mozzarella

Spritz a large sauté pan with nonstick cooking spray and place over medium heat. Add onion, tomato, turkey, and green pepper. Allow to cook 5 minutes, until soft. Add egg whites and salt and pepper to taste and stir. Allow to cook until the eggs are almost cooked through, then add the mozzarella. Keep on the heat until the cheese melts in. Serve immediately.

Snacks, Sides, and Other Anytime Favorites

Snacking, as we know, can be the enemy—but not if you're serving the right kinds of snacks and monitoring quantities. We like to have healthy snacks handy all the time, so that no one is tempted to eat junk when they're in the mood for a treat. Our healthy snacks have essentially become our treats, and believe it or not, by simply revamping how your family snacks, you are beginning to make some critical changes in the big picture of their nutrition.

Sweet Potato Fries

Prep Time: 1 hour 15 minutes
Serves 4

3 large sweet potatoes, peeled and cut lengthwise into strips about 4 inches long and $1/2$ inch thick
2 tablespoons olive oil
Salt and pepper
Leaves from 3 sprigs rosemary

Preheat oven to 425 degrees F. In a large bowl, toss the sliced sweet potatoes with olive oil and salt and pepper to taste, and place them on a nonstick cookie sheet. Sprinkle the rosemary leaves on top, and roast for 40 to 45 minutes, turning halfway through, until the sweet potatoes start to look slightly crispy and browned on the outside.

Bite-size Cheese Rolls
Prep Time: 10 minutes
Serves 2 to 4

2 slices turkey
2 slices ham
2 sticks mozzarella and cheddar blend string cheese
2 sticks organic, low-moisture, part-skim mozzarella string cheese
Crackers of your choice (whole wheat recommended)

Place turkey and ham slices flat on a cutting board. Place string cheese on top and roll up. Cut each roll into 4 bite-size pieces and hold together with colorful toothpicks. Place on a platter with crackers, serve, and enjoy.

Fruit Sticks

Prep Time: 15 minutes
Makes 8 skewers

1 organic apple such as sliced Pink Lady
1 banana, sliced
12 red seedless grapes
$\frac{1}{4}$ pound cantaloupe, sliced
$\frac{1}{4}$ pound strawberries

Arrange the fruit on 8 skewers, and let the kids make their own. Have fun with the order.

Sweet Grapes Snack

Prep Time: 5 minutes, plus chilling
Serves 1 to 2

20 seedless red grapes
3 teaspoons fat-free Cool Whip

Mix ingredients and chill.

Sweet Berries Snack

Prep Time: 5 minutes
Serves 2

$\frac{1}{2}$ cup diced strawberries
$\frac{1}{2}$ cup raspberries
$\frac{1}{2}$ cup blueberries
$\frac{1}{2}$ cup fat-free Cool Whip

Mix ingredients and chill.

Veggie Tree Snacks

Prep Time: 10 minutes
Serves 10

$1/2$ pound baby carrots
10 celery ribs, halved
$1/2$ pound raw broccoli florets
Fat-free ranch dressing for dipping

Simply chop or slice the veggies and assemble haphazardly with a toothpick in each one. Enjoy with ranch dressing or any other low-fat variety of your choice.

Whole Wheat Cinnamon French Toast Sticks

Prep Time: 20 minutes
Serves 2

$1/4$ cup skim milk
1 cup liquid egg whites
4 slices whole wheat cinnamon bread
Butter flavor nonstick cooking spray
Honey or light syrup

This is classic French toast done with a healthful twist. We use whole wheat cinnamon bread, which is already nice and sweet. In a dish with a flat bottom, whisk the skim milk with the egg whites, and soak the bread in the mixture for 10 minutes. Heat a large griddle over medium-high heat and spray with non-stick cooking spray. Add the egg-soaked bread and cook until golden, about 1 to 2 minutes per side. You can drizzle these with honey for an extra sweet kick, and cut the toasts into little sticks, which always makes it more fun for the kids.

The Veggie Edge

So many families today are leaning toward vegetarianism, and for very sound reasons, which include but are not limited to: significantly reduced rates of obesity, coronary heart disease, hypertension, type 2 diabetes, diet-related cancers, diverticular disease, constipation, and gallstones. An herbivorous diet can be lower in fat, clean, and endlessly nutritious. The real trick to its success is to understand the nature of variety when it comes to produce and to master the art of cleverly supplementing the diet with protein in other ways. Vegetarianism does not have to be a radical choice, either; you can certainly opt to have two out of three vegetarian nights per week and slowly wean your family into the appreciation of this time and these foods, which can be incredibly tasty if done right. We like to think of vegetarianism as a way to challenge yourself on a culinary level, finding interesting and creative ways of combining the freshest veggies to create fun family feasts forever.

If your household is vegan, remember that vitamin B_{12} is available only in animal protein, so you might consider taking B_{12} supplements, as a lack of this vitamin can lead to blood abnormalities, neurological problems, and impaired brain development. Please remember always to lay a proper nutritional foundation by first taking a good-quality, noncommercial-brand multivitamin before adding B₁₂. You should never just take a single B vitamin without providing a nice foundation of the entire B-vitamin family, which is what a good multivitamin will do. Otherwise, over the long-term, you can upset your B-vitamin balance.

Likewise, if you or any of the members of your family are lactose intolerant or simply don't love dairy products, remember that green, leafy veggies are also excellent sources of calcium. These veggies include kale, bok choy, mustard greens, and turnip greens. Many soy products also have added calcium. Finally, if meat is out of the question in your home, your family can get iron from dark leafy vegetables and whole grains.

Here are a few of our favorite vegetarian recipes.

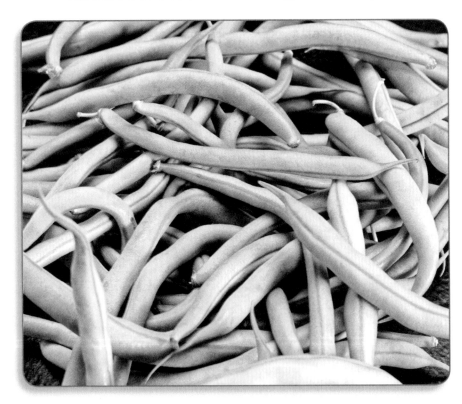

Spaghetti Squash with Soy Bolognese (aka Faux Bolognese)

Prep Time: 1 hour
Serves 4

1 (4- to 5-pound) spaghetti squash, halved
1 large onion, chopped
1$\frac{1}{2}$ tablespoon olive oil
1 garlic clove, chopped
2 large tomatoes, chopped
1 (2-ounce) package soy protein powder
Salt and pepper
1 tablespoon parsley, chopped
Grated Parmesan cheese (optional)

Preheat oven to 350 degrees F. Pour 1 cup water into an oven-safe baking dish and add the spaghetti squash halves, cut side down. Cover with foil and bake for 1 hour, or until soft. While the squash is in the oven, heat a large sauté pan over medium high heat. Add the onions and olive oil and cook until golden, stirring constantly. Add the garlic and cook for 2 minutes more. Reduce the heat to low and stir in the tomatoes. Cover and cook until a sauce forms, about 20 minutes. You can add a little tomato paste if you want more texture. Mix in the ground soy and season to taste. Cook for a few minutes until all the flavors blend, and keep on a very low heat.

Use a fork to shred the squash out of its shell into a large serving bowl. The flesh of the squash will come out in strings, hence the name *spaghetti squash*. Season to taste with salt and pepper. Serve the spaghetti squash with a ladleful of sauce on top, and sprinkle on some parsley and Parmesan cheese, if desired.

Eggplant Lasagna

Prep Time: 1 hour

Serves 8 to 10

5 large eggplants, cut lengthwise in $1/4$-inch-thick slices

$1/2$ cup olive oil, plus 2 teaspoons

Salt

3 large onions, chopped

3 cloves garlic, chopped

4 large tomatoes, chopped

1 (8-ounce) can tomato sauce

1 (6-ounce) can tomato paste

Pepper

1 pound low-fat, part-skim fresh mozzarella, sliced

Reduced-fat butter to grease the baking dish

Preheat oven to 375 degrees F. Brush the eggplant slices with $1/2$ cup of olive oil and sprinkle with salt. Place the slices in a single layer on baking sheets, taking care not to overlap them. Bake for 20 minutes, turning halfway through, until they are lightly golden. While the eggplants are roasting, heat a medium soup pot over medium heat. Add the remaining olive oil and onions. Cook, stirring frequently, until the onions begin to brown. Add the garlic and cook 1 minute more. Reduce the heat to low and add the tomatoes, tomato sauce, and tomato paste. Cover and cook 20 to 25 minutes, until the tomatoes are soft and have formed a sauce. Season to taste with salt and pepper.

Remove eggplant from oven and use a little bit of reduced-fat butter to grease a 9 by 12-inch baking dish for the lasagna. Arrange a flat layer of half of the eggplant slices, followed by a layer of half of the tomato sauce, spread evenly across on top. Then add a layer of half of the mozzarella. Repeat with the remaining eggplant, sauce, and cheese. Reduce the oven temperature to 350 degrees F and bake uncovered for 30 minutes, until the cheese is melted and bubbly.

Herbed Quinoa with Crushed Pistachios

Prep Time: 40 minutes
Serves 4 to 6

2 cups quinoa
2 tablespoons chopped dill
2 tablespoons chopped parsley
1 small onion, chopped
1 cup crushed pistachios
4 cups water (tip: substitute 2 cups of the water with chicken stock for added flavor)
Salt and pepper

Mix the quinoa, herbs, onion, pistachios, and water in pot and bring to a boil. Lower the heat, cover, and cook for about 30 minutes, or until the quinoa is cooked (you'll see its little sprout pop out from the grain when it's done). Season to taste with salt and pepper, and serve warm.

Kid-Friendly Smoothies for the Kid in Everyone

The key to creating healthy smoothies, according to nutritionist Suzanne Copp, MS, is to choose the purest ingredients possible. Organic milk, berries, yogurt, and peanut butter are ideal options. You can add a small amount of unflavored flax oil or MCT (medium chain triglycerides) oil to any of these. This will help make your shake frothier as well as healthier! You can also add xylitol (a sugar alcohol that is actually good for you) for desired sweetness. Instead of adding a sweetener, you can also try adding some vanilla extract for a change of taste.

Have fun experimenting! Everyone has different likes and dislikes when it comes to smoothies. Some like thicker drinks, others will prefer the smoother varieties. You can make this a fun family activity by letting everyone have a hand in building their own favorite smoothie concoctions.

Note: Mix all varieties in a blender. For smoothies that call for yogurt, Greek yogurt works best—it's very creamy, has higher protein content, and is less tart than other types. Smoothie recipes courtesy of Suzanne Copp, MS.

Berry Delight

Prep Time: 5 minutes
1 serving

$\frac{1}{2}$ cup plain yogurt
$\frac{1}{2}$ cup water
$\frac{1}{2}$ cup ice
1 cup frozen blueberries, strawberries, or cherries

Fresh Berry Blast

Prep Time: 5 minutes
Serves 1 to 2

1 cup organic, hormone-free whole milk
$\frac{1}{2}$ cup water
$\frac{1}{2}$ cup ice
$1\frac{1}{2}$ cup fresh blueberries, strawberries, raspberries, or a
mixture of all three
1 scoop plain or vanilla whey protein powder with no artificial
sweeteners (optional)

Banana-Choco Blast

Prep Time: 5 minutes
Serves 1

$\frac{1}{2}$ cup plain yogurt
$\frac{1}{2}$ cup water
$\frac{1}{2}$ cup ice
1 frozen banana
1 scoop chocolate whey protein powder or 2–3 tablespoons
unsweetened cocoa powder

Banana-Cinnamon Blast

Prep Time: 5 minutes

Serves 1

½ cup plain yogurt

½ cup water

½ cup ice

1 frozen banana

1 teaspoon cinnamon

Coconut-Chocolate Infusion

Prep Time: 5 minutes

Serves 1

½ cup plain yogurt

½ cup water

½ cup ice

½ cup coconut milk

1 scoop chocolate whey protein powder or 3 tablespoons
unsweetened cocoa powder

1–2 tablespoons unsweetened shredded coconut (optional)

Peanut Butter–Chocolate Smoothie

Prep Time: 5 minutes

Serves 1

1 cup organic chocolate milk

1 cup ice

1–2 tablespoons organic peanut butter

1 scoop chocolate whey protein powder or 3 tablespoons
unsweetened cocoa powder

Healthy (Essential!) Tips for the Whole Family

Here are some other core basics that we like to stick to as a crew, some fundamental little bits of truth that we feel have the power to guide a life of real wellness. Our hope is to remind you gently of their importance. These are likely principles that you have heard before, so we know we are not reinventing the wheel. We hope you can remember to keep them in your radar of awareness, and better yet, impart them, with love, to your own families.

MO' H₂O

We have all heard that one of the basic rules of health is to drink plenty of water, but we know that remembering to do so can be tricky, and for some people, drinking water is an absolute chore. But because proper hydration is unequivocally important, especially if we are going to be physically active (which we are), we must think about how to get our families hydrated, *water or not*. Remember: the key is to be resourceful.

- **Make Ice Pops** Get some cute-shaped ice trays and freeze some (low-sugar) fruit juice diluted with water in each slot. Everyone loves an ice pop. Especially a cute-shaped one. Especially on a hot summer day.

- **Water Cooler** If you can, consider investing in a freestanding water cooler, so everyone has open access to it and can have a cup of water without even thinking about it.

- **The Melons** Start thinking about recipes with foods like cucumber, melons, and watermelons that are high in water content, as well as foods like homemade chicken soup.

MANY SMALL MEALS

We have all been conditioned, for whatever reason, to believe that eating three large meals a day is the way to allocate feeding times and quantities. It is an ancient paradigm of consumption that has essentially ruled our understanding of food: breakfast, lunch, and dinner—that is what we know. But, as many of you probably also know, research now shows that eating five or six smaller meals a day is an even more efficient way to run the body, so to speak, and happens besides to be a fantastic way to get your family to start thinking about snacking *smart*. Teach your children from the get-go about the benefits of choosing small meal items such as turkey slices with hummus and celery sticks with peanut butter. Explain to them that by eating smaller quantities a few times throughout the day, they will have increased energy to keep their "furnaces burning and alive," never allowing their metabolisms to get sluggish. Here is a list of smart snacks that you can always throw into your beach bag or purse or have around at home.

Smart Snacks

Almonds

Carrot sticks with a squeeze of lemon

Celery sticks with peanut butter

Dried fruit

Low-fat string cheese

Low-fat yogurts and cottage cheese

Fruits, especially in season

Edamame

Low-sugar fruit sorbets

Homemade trail mix

Fruit smoothies

Soy chips

Low-fat cheese and whole wheat crackers

Turkey slices dipped in hummus

Hard-boiled eggs

Whole wheat crackers with avocado and lemon juice

Scoop of tuna salad

Apples slices with peanut butter

Sliced bananas and peanut butter on whole wheat toast

Sliced bananas with a scoop of low-fat cottage cheese

Sliced pears with a wedge of low-fat hard cheese of your choice

Grapes with low-fat hard cheese of your choice

Cup of homemade chicken soup (make one batch and sip it all week)

Half a whole wheat English muffin with low-fat cheese

GOOD MORNING, SUNSHINE

Make breakfast matter . . . because it *does*. So many studies have shown that having breakfast not only gives the necessary kick-start to the metabolism each morning but also provides the necessary nourishment for the day and, for children especially, gives the necessary nutrition to perform at one's peak capacity. Plus, it gives the family a chance to sit together at the top of the morning, when you can share news and talk about the day to come. We strongly believe that every opportunity to sit and eat with your family is a unique chance to connect as a group. Take advantage of these precious moments, make them a part of the collective routine, and all the while know that these little details are precisely the ones that will make an impact on the physical and mental wellness of the people you love most.

EAT TO PLAY

We always find that one of the best ways to teach our kids is by making everything a *game*. Start by not taking yourself so seriously, and dare to have fun with the day-to-day. For example, one night a week, hold a Food Trivia game, where you come up with questions about nutrition, and award the winner with a healthy treat of their choice. Make up cards with questions like "Which is the healthiest protein of the following three: bacon, grilled chicken, or steak," or "Name a good fat and name a bad fat," and have a point system for right answers. Keep it playful, but make sure the message is clear: that the joy of eating comes with the responsibility of knowing *how to eat right*.

Another fun idea is to have a Blind Date night, where you blindfold your kids and have them guess what they are eating, all for the sake of really tasting and experiencing food from an even more profound sensory perspective. Call it A Night of Tastings, and have everyone try to describe what they are savoring, how their taste buds are experiencing the process of food in this bizarre but intimate way. It gets everyone excited about the possibilities of food, and also gets everyone in the mode of *appreciation,* which is key in the mastery of relating to food.

Simple little activities such as mixing up some homemade lemonade together or making a giant fruit salad as a group can help shape the collective mission to eat healthy foods and at the same time enjoy one another's company. Even tiny little modifications will enhance the experience, like having more meals outside on your porch or in your backyard, where the sounds of nature can be the backdrop to your meal, as opposed to the endless ringing of cell phones and incoming text messages. Commit to once-a-week BBQ night, and once a week to have a group breakfast under the sky. Dare to revitalize your own sense of creativity by coming up with ideas that will keep all the nutrients coming, along with great times and memories to be shared by all.

THE TREAT BEAT

A quick note on treats and indulgences. We know very well that everyone's got to live a little—so the occasional treat now and again is not going to be something we condemn. In fact, we highly encourage that your family take part in everything, try everything, and taste everything—but always with the spirit of balance, awareness, and moderation in mind. Everyone has their own particular soft spot: for some people it comes in the form of white chocolate, and for others it will be a fresh hot croissant. These "soft spots," however, should never be confused with straight-up junk food, that processed garbage that comes in little bags and leaves your kids' fingers a frightening shade of orange. You know exactly what we're talking about. Think, instead, about treats in their most classical sense: an ice cream cone, a piece of good chocolate, or an oatmeal raisin cookie. Redefine the family sense of what a treat is, and start introducing a new world of treats—one that includes a serious connection to nutrition and wellness.

Rethink Your Treats

Instead of . . .	Have or Serve . . .
Ice cream	Frozen yogurt or sorbet
Potato chips	Soy chips
Chocolate	Cacao nibs
Pizza	Tomato soup with low-fat cheese
Brownies	Oat bran raisin muffins
Chocolate chip cookie	Oatmeal raisin cookie
Chocolate milk	Almond milk
Candy	Frozen grapes or dried fruit like apricots, dates, figs, mangoes, and apples
Gummy bears	Fresh lychees
Hamburger	Veggie, turkey, salmon, or chicken burger on a whole wheat bun
French fries	Sweet potato fries

Instead of . . .	Have or Serve . . .
Lasagna	Eggplant lasagna (see recipe, page 88)
Bacon	Turkey or soy bacon
Sausage	Chicken or soy sausage
Ham	Lean turkey breast
Fried chicken	Oven-baked crispy chicken
Fried chicken sandwich	Grilled chicken in whole wheat pita
BLT	Turkey or soy bacon, lettuce, and tomato on whole wheat toast
Mozzarella sticks	Low-fat string cheese
Fried shrimp	Shrimp Provençal
Fried calamari	Grilled calamari
White rice	Quinoa or brown rice
Macaroni and cheese	Whole wheat macaroni with low-fat cheese
Chocolate mousse	Almond butter
Grilled cheese	Low-fat grilled cheese on whole-grain bread
Apple pie	Baked apples with raisins and cinnamon
Banana split	Lightly baked bananas with cinnamon
Milk shake	Fruit smoothie
Sweetened cereal	Oatmeal with nuts and raisins
Mashed potatoes	Sweet potato mash
Clam chowder	Whole wheat linguine with clams, olive oil, lemon, parsley, and salt
Lollipops	Fruit juice ice pops
French toast	Whole wheat French toast with fruit
Waffles and cream	Whole-grain waffles and fat-free Cool Whip
Pancakes	Whole-grain pancakes with fruit
Eggs and toast	Scrambled egg whites with whole grain toast

Instead of . . .	Have or Serve . . .
Eggs Benedict	Poached egg on a lightly buttered whole grain English muffin and a side of turkey bacon
Ham and cheese	Turkey slices and avocado on whole-grain bread
Bagel and cream cheese	Whole wheat pita with hummus
Hot dog	Turkey or soy dog on a whole wheat bun
Nachos and cheese	Whole-grain tortilla chips with low-fat cheese and avocado
Cashews	Almonds
Chips and dip	Veggie sticks and fat-free ranch dressing
Candy bar	Low-fat whole-grain energy bar
Store-bought juice	Freshly squeezed juice
Corn dog	Grilled polenta with wild mushrooms and herbs
Sloppy Joe	Seasoned ground soy protein on a whole wheat bun
Pop-Tarts	Whole wheat toast with fig spread
Potato skins	Baked sweet potato with low-fat cheese
Chow mein	Soba (buckwheat) noodles with sautéed vegetables
Fried rice	Brown rice sautéed with soy sauce, eggs, and vegetables
Cupcakes	Bran muffins with raisins
Sweetened licorice	Dried fruit
Cheese fries	Half a sweet potato with low-fat melted cheese

We hope we have in some way inspired you to loosen some of your preconceived ideas about proper nutrition and expanded your understanding of the art of experiencing food as a family.

We sincerely wish for you that your table always abounds with delicious, nutritious meals, memorable moments, and all kinds of quality time.

And it is exactly in the spirit of quality time that we are ready to move on to the other fundamental element of our campaign toward health—*family fitness*. In the section that follows, we will step out of our kitchens and dining rooms and into the world, where we explore the nature of physical activity in the context of pure, unbridled, unstoppable, good old-fashioned *fun*.

Fun
Family
Fitness

The Art of Taking

the "Work" out of

"Working Out"

Our relationship as a couple was in many ways shaped by sports; after all, we met for the very first time on a softball field. One of us needed a glove, and the other, wouldn't you know, conveniently had one in the car. Many years later, we held our first date in a bowling alley; the third date was on a racquet-ball court. We would become fierce Ping-Pong opponents and stretching buddies all at once, and our five-year wedding anniversary was celebrated with a volleyball tournament, replete with teams and scores and food and trophies, and games that lingered late into the night. And so it would continue for the rest of our lives as a couple, and today as parents, our energy as a group is always fueled by the spirit of healthy competition.

For many, however, the concept of exercise or working out kicks in only with middle age, just as panic is about to really set in with the quickly aging self. This angst-ridden panic shows up around the time when belly fat starts to develop a life of its own, arms begin to sag, and the notion of climbing a flight of stairs becomes the worst thought imaginable. That's when many of us abruptly snap out of our laze, reluctantly join the gym, force ourselves to do the dreaded crunches, chug water like thirsty savages, and entertain diets named after trendy neighborhoods in popular vacation cities. We hastily lose ten wretched pounds, subsisting on grilled chicken (white meat only) and salad without dressing for two weeks, and then a month later gain it all back, because we felt deprived to begin with, and so consoled our void with all varieties of sugared confections and other doughy yummies. We stupidly put our trust in fad diets that force one to abstain from this or that

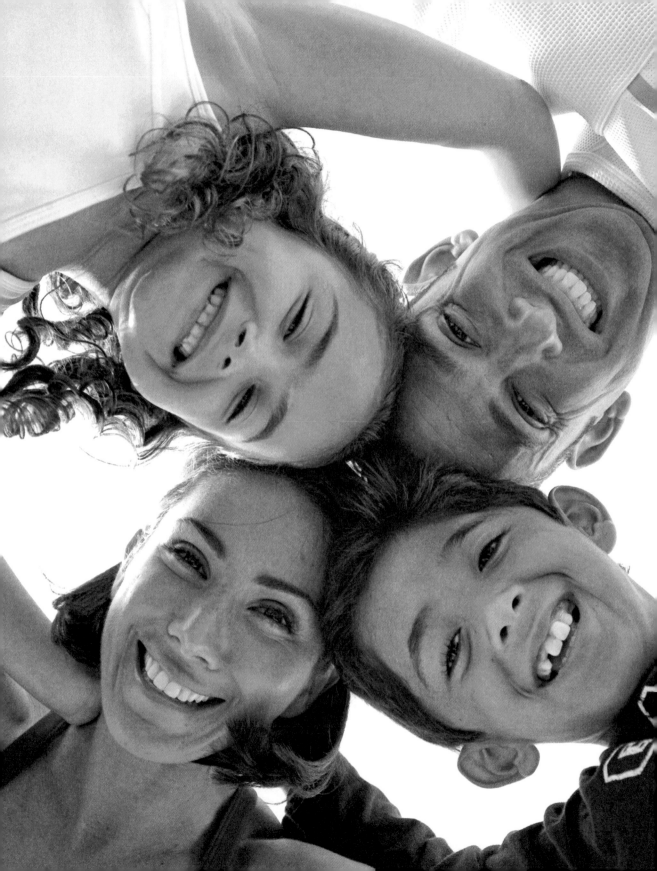

taboo product, be it sugar or carbs, and then we miss these things so incredibly that we end up eating more of them and gaining back more weight than we had before the whole thing started. On the other end of this dark spectrum are those of us who stop eating altogether, naively thinking that starving ourselves will lead to some fatless reality, and in that delusion, we may develop all varieties of eating disorders, which is also not a pretty picture, much less if we have kids around watching our behavior and learning our ways.

People, does it have to be this ugly? Perhaps it does for some of us grown-ups, who are fixed in our ways and just don't know any better. But as far as our children go, well, it's another story entirely, and being able to instill the right kinds of fitness and food habits in your family from the start conditions them for a life less agonized than perhaps yours was regarding self-discipline and body image—and it also puts *you,* as parents, into the mind-set of activity, mobility, and initiative. Isn't that precisely what we all need a little more of in our lives? What we would like to propose here is not only a sense of discipline but also a sense of balance, because, unlike those aforementioned fad diets, the lifestyle we're talking about here is a lasting one, one with staying power, that you can practice safely all of the time, forever.

As serious athletes, who define our happiness by the quality of our physical health, we would like to offer you a possibility that is far less anxiety-laden than the scenario posed above, one that will suit you whether you are an adult or a child. We would like to offer you the possibility of a world where the scope and range of "exercise" is enormously expanded; where activities that promote fitness become one and the same with *quality family time;* and where the process and practice of fitness are taught to your kids right from the start, empowering you with the ability to create a collectively healthy and active family. Burn calories and make memories at the same time!

The problem, as we see it, is that kids are exposed to so much that is *not healthy* for them, or even *not healthy enough*, and become conditioned to subsist on some kind of mediocre paradigm of nutrition that ultimately turns them into lazy, semi-out-of-shape adults. Maybe some of that would be diminished slightly if kids had a new conception of what exercise could mean—or if they could be gently conned into mobility through the advent of different types of activities than the ones they are used to. Because of how much stimulation children receive today from the technological world alone, so much about being a living, physical, human body is getting lost in the alluring prospect of lying on a couch while lost in some virtual reality. Or our kids are like those high-tech employees laboring at computer desks all day, which is also horrible for their developing bodies, which need to bend and stretch and move and, most important, *be in the world*. The advent of computers and video games of course has its positives, but in general, we believe that children should be encouraged to play outside, engage in games and sports, and have the desire to maximize their time of recreation with active, stimulating activities that simultaneously move their bodies and their minds.

It all begins with a basic shift in attitude, not unlike the one we made regarding food, and it must stem from the essential group commitment to *become more active*. This means not only that you literally have to *do* more; it also means you all have to start getting creative about *what* you do. We would like to believe that this new element of "planning and programming" will get you more jazzed about doing your exercise, as this challenge will make the whole endeavor of staying active way more playful, personal, customized, and fun. Besides all that, it will engender a sense of unity with the members of your clan, who will have no choice but to strengthen their bond as they collectively embark on what will hopefully be a dynamic, energetic, on-the-go, always stimulating campaign for health. Being together feels good. Doing the right things for your body feels good. What could be better than doing both at once?

In the same way that buying the right ingredients when you go food shopping ensures that your family will eat the right kinds of meals, the same rule applies with fitness and exercise: if you provide the right kinds of ideas for activities and back them up by being ready with all the safety equipment and relevant gear, the family remains permanently poised to *do* . . . and *doing* is exactly what this section is all about.

In the pages that follow, you will find a wide range of ideas for activities, games, sports, and exercises; there are suggestions for things to do, whether you are at home, on a trip, at the beach, in the pool, in your backyard, on the slopes, in the woods . . . pretty much anywhere, anytime. These tips comprise our own family's way of spending time the way we believe it is most meaningful: by treating our bodies right, by being one with nature as often as possible, and by being together as often as possible. As parents, the demands of both of our careers make every second that we have with our children sacred and special; more to the point, because our time is so limited, we are aware that we also have to make the best use of it, milking every second to move, to inspire, to teach, to do, and *to enjoy* with our family.

I remember as a kid in Puerto Rico, our parents used to take us to El Yunque, which is one of the largest and most impressive tropical rainforests in the world. There, we would excitedly scour the area for these delicious little wild berries that we would devour just as excitedly as we had found them. The whole thing became a little game, everyone competing for the largest arsenal of berries. The whole plan was at once dynamic and fun—and kept us all in the groove of actively enjoying Mother Nature's greatest bounty. The process of picking these gorgeous, tangy berries out there in the jungle connected us deeply to our stunning surroundings, and gave us a primal sense of what it means to be a human being on this planet.

—*Laura Posada*

For us it has always been vital to teach our children about the merits of being leaders and the difference between being the kind of person who wants to be a leader, and works for it, and the kind who sits back, waiting for things to happen. We tell our children the true stories of our own childhoods, when we were not necessarily the best at the sports and activities that we took part in—but we were always the ones who worked the hardest. We have always explained to our kids that success is not going to come knocking on their doors, and that life is their chance *to create their own successes*. We teach them about the importance of being survivors, just like the ones on the television program, who work with all of their might to come out on top, proving the idea that, indeed, only the strong survive.

Of course, when they are young, sometimes it's hard for them to understand fully the importance of such ideals, but slowly, gradually, you teach them, and they catch on. It starts with the basics, like explaining to them the importance of excelling at school and of learning how to do things for yourself—because from the time they were babies, they were used to having everything done by you. If you teach them to *want* to be independent winners and doers, as they evolve into their own realities of independence, they become naturally poised to succeed.

THE D LIST

Growing up, we knew a coach, a real character, who used four words to guide our motivation: *DRIVE, DEDICATION, DISCIPLINE, DESIRE.* The Four Ds, the coach called them. Those words always sat close to home with both of us, as livers of athletic lives and believers in the power of fitness. Over the years, we have taken the liberty of adding to that list of Ds.

DECIDE	*DREAM*
DRIVE	*DEFINE*
DANCE	*DOMINATE*
DEVELOP	*DIVINE*
DEFY	*DO*
DEVOTE	*DEMAND*
DELIVER	*DESIGNATE*
DARE	*DICTATE*
DIRECT	*DETERMINATION*

We take those words with us to our work and to our workouts, but most important, we *live* them right at home, where our son and daughter can learn by example, and share, with us, in the joy of being strong and fit. Sometimes a single word can have great potency, and by simply reminding ourselves of these powerful little minislogans, by repeating them in our minds, we can empower ourselves with the good stuff. And don't forget, when we are empowered, we are capable of anything.

All it takes is a little creativity about how to make your plans, and fortunately for us, Mother Nature herself has simplified the planning, giving us four seasons, which are the fundamental blueprint for all activities. Later, we will see how the different times of year can directly dictate which activities will be best to plan, and how keeping to the rhythm of nature is a beautiful way to maximize the time and energy spent on fitness and family time.

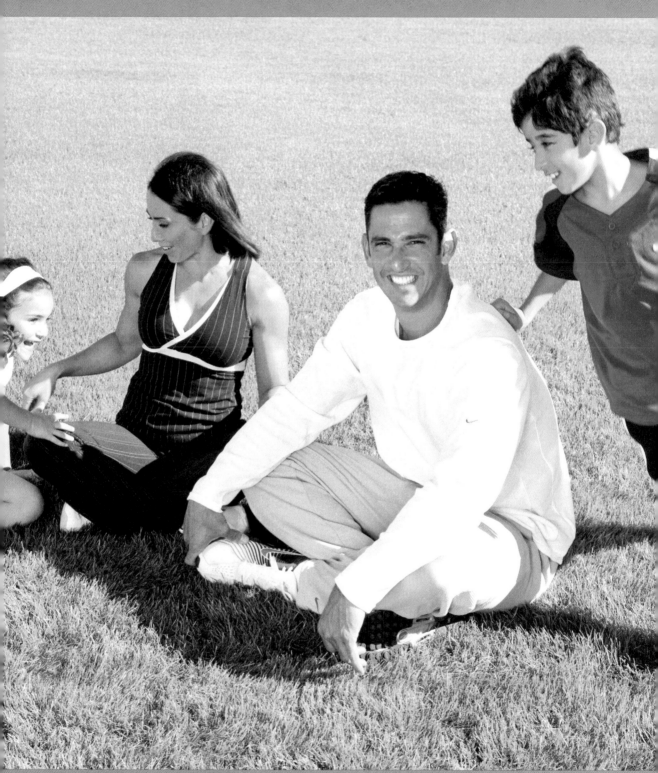

Healthy Body = Healthy Mind = Healthy Spirit

First, let's get back to basics for a minute. What is the big deal about fitness and exercise? Well, besides the very obvious, such as health (not to beat a dead horse already)—there is a subtler list of internal virtues that comes with the pursuit of a healthy body; elements that also exist in our *inner world,* that can only serve us well, as humans trying to be the best they can be.

Some people might believe that the athletic types are just that—athletic. But guess what? The virtues of athleticism go far beyond the physical realm and into other, less tangible, more nuanced areas of experience. The truth is that the pursuit and performance of athletic activities do as much for our brains as they do for brawn, and being aware of these benefits helps to rev up our gusto on the road to optimal fitness and health. Think of it this way: all of the attributes on the following Hot List may or may not work on the various muscles you can feel in your body, but consider that they work even harder on the invisible muscle of our *integrity*—which empowers us as people, in sports, and in life.

As you go through the list, try to remember the words being described. Hold them close, and really know them. Remember the power of single words and the potency in always reminding yourself about their core meanings. Share these words with the members of your family. Remind everyone that these words exist, what they mean, and more important, what they can mean. Instead of talking over lunch about celebrity gossip or the latest video game releases, consider having a conversation about, say, *balance*. Ask your kids if they know what it is. Make them guess if they don't. Jump-start their curiosities about the very things they will be working with during this new program of *doing*. See it as a full-spectrum approach to the Fit Home Challenge, whereby the family works on itself, from the inside out. And remember, for every attribute that you think you or someone in your family needs work on, there are always solutions that can help take you or anyone else in the right direction. Let's take a look.

THE FITNESS HOT LIST

Commitment

Commitment is the little switch that we hit in our hearts and minds when we summon up the will to do something. Not only that, commitment is also the energy that allows us to see our goals right to the end. Commitment holds us steady and resolute toward the finish line, fueled by our desire to do what we set out to do. Commitment is what we need to refine that which matters to us most.

> **TIP:** If you feel you lack commitment, decide right now to practice something every day. It could be dancing, singing, running, biking, whatever naturally comes to mind. Commit to doing this activity every single day, no matter what. Sometimes it helps to do the activity at the same time every day, to work on your sense of routine, and in time, you will see that your "commitment" has somehow paid off.

Endurance

Endurance is the fire inside us that burns with our sheer will and determination. It is the force of our true potential hard at work, and it is one of those virtues that play as importantly in the game of fitness as in the game of life. When we master the art of endurance, we enter the realm of being true survivors. In this space of victory, we can tap into what it means to be a winner. There's no getting around it: winners endure.

> **TIP:** If you feel you lack endurance, practice a cardio-vascular activity, such as treading water in the swimming pool or light jogging, and time yourself each time you have a session. See if you can break your own record every single day in order to work constantly on your endurance. Keep a written record of your progress so that you have a tangible account of your success and potential.

Flexibility

We like to take this word literally as well as metaphorically. Being flexible is a true merit, all athletics aside. Flexible, after all, means adaptable, malleable, elastic, and *able to move*. Aren't these traits that we want as we navigate through this complex world? Being flexible arms us with a sense of possibility and a sense of openness; it keeps our bodies and minds in a constant state of reception.

> **TIP:** If you feel you lack flexibility, consider joining a beginner's yoga class, which is a safe and excellent way to explore new edges of your flexibility. Learning how to breathe while you stretch is a fundamental way to home in on the potential of stretching and the depths to which you can go with your muscles in a relaxed, deep-breathing state. Flexibility is a lot about letting go, letting freshly oxygenated blood flow freely through the body, and about making sure to send enough air into the body, by breathing, to make sure that can happen as efficiently as possible.

Coordination

Being coordinated means you can multitask; it means you have control over your body and you own that control with a sense of balance and confidence. To be coordinated is to be fully connected to your mind, limbs, faculties, and senses in a comprehensive way. Sports are a great way to develop coordination, a skill that carries beautifully into all other aspects of life.

> **TIP:** If you feel you lack coordination, consider joining a dance class of your choice, which will undoubtedly help to hone your coordination, your sense of rhythm, and your ability to direct your body in sync with a group. There are all kinds of dance styles, including hip-hop, salsa, jazz, modern, ballet, tap, swing, tango, and more. So take your pick, and put on your dancing shoes.

Motivation

Motivation is our "inner push," the silent nudge within that compels us toward our goals, an undercurrent of fuel that feeds our desire to succeed. We need motivation to accomplish things, be they on the field, on the job, or anywhere else in life where things *need to happen;* without motivation, we are like cars out of gas. Cultivating a sense of motivation early in a child's life helps him to tap into his own God-given talents and resources to achieve success.

> **TIP:** If motivation is your issue, consider starting your mornings by repeating a daily mantra, something inspiring that you tell yourself and that you know deep down will help spark the fire of motivation. Try something like "It is my duty to do everything I can to be the best I can be." Consider saying the mantra as a group to rev up the collective energy, which is also an excellent way to stir up the energy of motivation.

Stamina

Our stamina is our power source. It is like our endurance, but it is more than that—it feeds our endurance. The stronger our stamina, the more endurance we can demonstrate, which ultimately means we are sturdy and capable. Though stamina is in many ways physical, it is also very much a mental thing. Through the power of determination, one can learn to develop stamina.

> **TIP:** If you're the kind of person who clocks out and doesn't stay in the game, working on your stamina will be a great opportunity to practice the art of fortitude. Stamina goes hand in hand with endurance, and you'll want to cultivate both if you want to be a winner. To work on your stamina, try to stay very alert in the moment that you feel like giving up, and force yourself in that moment to give just a little bit more. It does not have to be loads more—just enough to prove to yourself that you are able. Take your cue from Obama, and say, "Yes I can!"

Circulation

Blood flow is life force, and the more freely it flows, the more open our bodies are to the prospect of total wellness, as the high-speed oxygenated blood reaches all of our muscles and internal organs, not the least of which are the heart and brain. Proper circulation is vital to good health, and we should always find ways to improve it by stretching and deep breathing, in an effort to send high-speed oxygenated blood to all our different parts.

> **TIP:** If you feel you have poor circulation, whether a medical expert has told you so or you just feel it on your own, activities like yoga and swimming are wonderful ways to work the circulatory system. Needless to say, if you have a persistent medical issue, you should be consulting with your doctor.

Determination

Determination is the arrow of perseverance that shoots us from point A to point B; it is sheer will, wearing its favorite outfit and ready to rock the world of our goals. Without determination, we lack desire, and without desire, we are burned-out candles, darkened and purposeless. Determination gives us purpose.

> **TIP:** If your sense of determination seems off, try to identify exactly what your goals are. Think about the ones you want most, ask yourself what you will have to do to achieve them—be they in sports or in life—and imagine that it is your sheer determination that will help you accomplish them.

Performance

Performance is showtime; it is our chance to shine, show the world what we are made of, and give our all. When we perform, we call on the powers of our skill, talent, and perseverance to come out on top. And when we perform well, we come out right on top.

> **TIP:** If you're the kind of person who gets performance anxiety and crumbles when it's showtime, the best medicine is very simple: deep breathing. When we take deep, full breaths into our bellies (instead of our chests), we calm the nervous system and regulate our own heart rates—both of which will likely quell the stress of having to "perform." So next time you're on, take a few deep breaths, and let the exhalations fuel your performance.

Strength

Strength is power, and power is ability. Cultivating an identity of strength, be it physical or mental, we believe, is paramount to living a truly conscious and examined life. In fact, we don't separate between physical and mental strength—to us, they are inextricably linked, they are one.

> **TIP:** Some people simply do not feel strong—be it physically or mentally—a deficiency that can cause many varieties of problems in life. Strength is critical, and if you feel yours is lacking, you must look inside to the places within that you know empower you—your talents, your blessings, your charm, whatever it may be for you—and allow yourself to feel the strength of that empowerment. In a nutshell: force yourself to tap into your natural, God-given strength. It's there; you just have to believe it.

Balance

Balance allows us to stand up straight, but make no mistake about it—balance is also very much a mental thing. With balance, there is calm; with balance there is effortlessness; with balance there is control—some of the basic elements of truly positive experiences.

> **TIP:** If you feel you lack balance, again, yoga does wonders. After all, yoga is all about the balance between mind, body, and spirit; its postures elicit both a physical and mental approach to balance. Think of it as one-stop shopping.

Sportsmanship

We spoke about it before, but there's no reason to leave it off our Hot List. This is where the power of group dynamics comes alive, where we can play at the edges of healthy competition, keeping to a high standard of ethics and integrity. Sportsmanship teaches us about coexistence and compassion, and puts us, at eye level, in the face of opposition, which we must balance with goodwill.

> **TIP:** If you feel you need to work on your sense of sportsmanship, try the simple exercise of always putting yourself in the other person's shoes. Imagine how they might feel if they won, or if they lost, and try to relate to both cases in your own way. Basically, try to be more conscious of the feelings that arise with winning and losing, and always keep them in the back of your mind.

Stress Relief

There is no getting around the fact that exercise relieves stress. Perhaps it is something about the elevated heart rate, the sweat, the deep breathing, and the repetition of movements that moves the mind from a state of frenzy and tension to a place of loosening and opening. Moving the body essentially moves the mind—and very often, the mind needs just that kind of nudge to be wrestled from the pestering grasp of thoughts, cravings, aversions, and fears.

> **TIP:** This one is critical and, for many people, possibly also the most challenging idea to put into practice. Stress dominates many of us, paralyzing our ability to function in our own lives, afflicting us mentally, which inevitably affects us physically. Think about the pain in your back or neck right now, and you'll know exactly what we are talking about. To relieve stress, there is a lot you can do, and the key is to find what works for you. Some people might explore meditation, which is known to reduce stress and foster a sense of balance. Yoga has the same kinds of benefits, with the added incentive of also helping to relieve the physical stress in the body. Singing and dancing might be another way to shatter the hold of stress. It's a matter of knowing yourself, knowing what makes you happy and calm, and doing it. A lot.

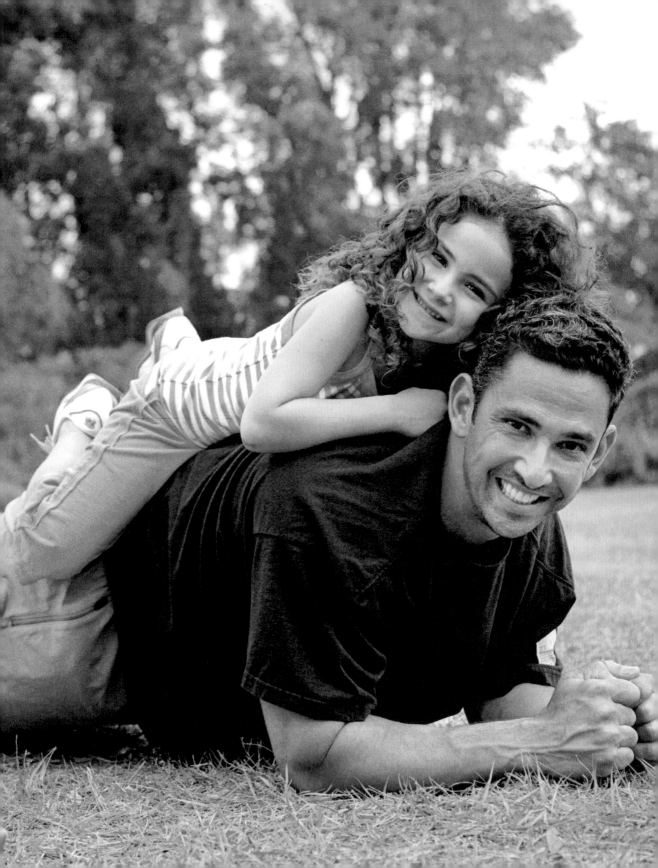

Quality Time

Last, but certainly not least, is quality time—to us it is actually the most important concept. In this day and age, where there is such a high volume of outside stimulation for our kids, when they are so caught up with the quickly changing world around them, there is so little time and energy left for family time. And family time, the way we see it, is the joy of living. Planning fun activities with your children tells them that you are all buddies, that the mission is unity, and that you are one. It shows them, by example, about the virtues of enjoying life and of making the best use of one's time and energy.

> **TIP:** If you feel that your family does not get enough quality time, consider revamping the rules in your house about activities such as TV watching and video game playing. We encourage you to use this book as a source of inspiration and guide for fun ideas, and get everyone excited about hanging out and having a good time.

KNOW YOUR NUMBERS

As you embark on this crusade of fitness, it will be essential to teach your kids about things like *heart rate* and *pulse*. You will want them to be able to check their levels of cardiovascular success, according to how hard they are supposed to be working. Explain to children that their pulse is their heart rate—the number of times their heart beats in one minute. Help them understand that their pulse is lower when they are at rest and increases when they exercise (because more oxygen-rich blood is needed by the body at this time). Make sure they get the idea that knowing how to take your pulse can help you evaluate your exercise program. A quick reading of one's own pulse can often tell if one needs to push harder or hold back.

There are other things to consider when you exercise, such as *maximum heart rate,* which is the highest heart rate achieved during maximal exercise; and there is *target heart rate,* the zone where you gain the most benefits of your exercise. You can calculate each person's maximum heart rate with this simple equation: 220 - age = predicted maximum heart rate. You usually reach your target heart rate when your exercise heart rate (pulse) is 60 to 80 percent of your maximum heart rate. This, of course, will vary from person to person, but as parents it is your duty to know everyone's numbers and encourage everyone to constantly push their own abilities.

Another number to consider is everyone's BMI, or body mass index, the formula that doctors use to estimate how much body fat a person has, based on his or her weight and height. The BMI formula uses height and weight measurements to calculate a BMI number. For kids, BMI is plotted on a growth chart that uses percentile lines to tell whether a child is underweight, healthy weight, overweight, or obese. Different BMI charts are used for boys and girls under the age of twenty, because the amount of body fat differs between boys and girls and because body fat changes as kids grow. To measure your child's BMI, you'll need an accurate height and weight measurement. The best way to get accurate measurements is by having kids weighed and measured at a doctor's office or at school.

STRETCHING

Growing up, we didn't love stretching; it was one of those things we had to be forced to do, as a matter of safety, but we certainly didn't welcome it. Today we wish we had been more enthusiastic about stretching and had done it with more heart, given the positive effect it can have on the overall well-being of your body, and because it is hard to start stretching for the first time when you're forty. Besides being excellent for general well-being, stretching is also a fantastic way to kick off *all* of your activities. Think about it this way: this is a wonderful habit to instill in your kids while they are young (and inherently more flexible), as it is no secret that stretching before exercise is the healthy, safe, and correct way to approach one's physical fitness. If they start stretching as children, they will not only be more flexible in the long run but, more important, they will develop awareness about the importance of properly taking care of their bodies.

Following are some suggestions and notes for basic stretches that are OK for kids. Before they even begin stretching, encourage them to do a few jumping jacks or run around

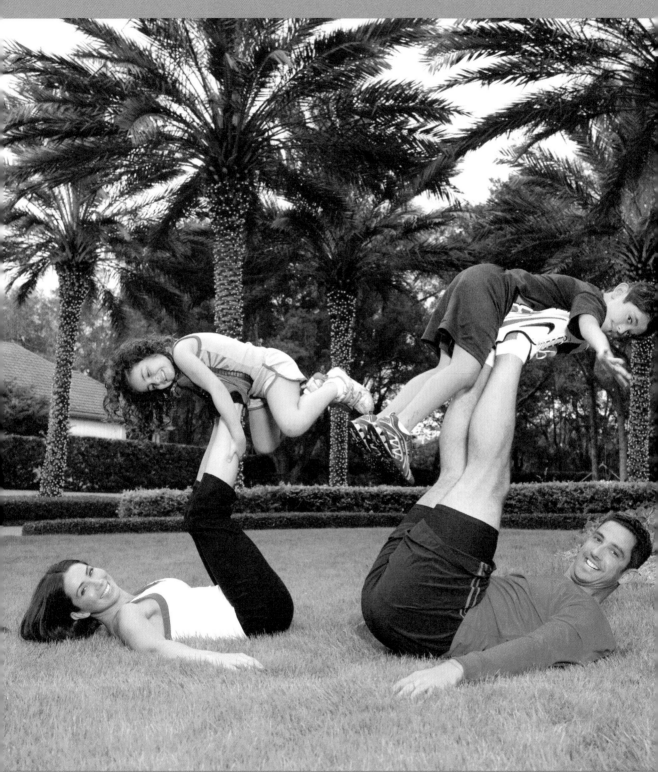

a bit, just to get the heart pumping. You could opt to focus on seated stretches, as it is often too challenging for kids to juggle balancing and stretching. Remaining seated allows them to release fully into the stretch and gradually relax into the tight muscles.

Alternatively, if your kids are up for it, you can opt to start in a standing position and work your way down from the head to the feet. If you choose this way, start by gently rolling the head around in circular motions until the neck feels nice and loose. You can move the stretch down to your waist and move that part around, also in circular motions, until the torso starts to open up. Then swing your arms from the shoulders backward and forward until the upper body starts to loosen and open.

Then stand straight up with feet and toes touching, and bend from the waist down, with as straight a spine as possible, to reach for your toes. You can start by touching your fingertips to the ground, and gradually move on to your knuckles, or even the whole palm. If your palms touch, you are ready to touch your nose to your knees for a fantastic, comprehensive, 360-degree stretch. You can also do just the basic posture of sitting with your legs stretched out before you, belly tucked in and back held straight, trying to reach for your toes. Remember to keep your spine as straight as possible and to take deep breaths into the belly, and then reach harder on the exhale. You will feel this stretch all along the backs of your legs, and even into the lower and upper back, which will also lengthen downward.

Another stretch you can do is to stand with legs at hips' distance apart, and bend from the waist down, holding your

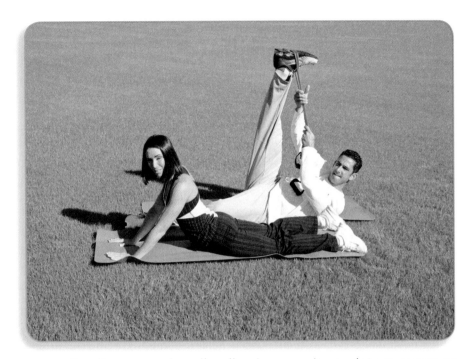

opposite elbows, and really allowing gravity to let your upper body dangle downward. Take very deep inhalations in this position, and with each slow exhalation, allow the upper body to weigh down even more, closer to the ground. Touch one foot with both hands, and hold there; and then touch the other foot, and hold there. You can then touch each hand to the opposite foot, and twist and reach up with the other arm straight behind you into the air. Do this on both sides, as with all exercises, for better symmetry of the body. You'll see that this series is fantastic to open up the upper back, which becomes a sore spot for a lot of us as we get older. By learning how to keep the shoulder belt relaxed when we're young, we can hope for more flexible, less painful shoulders in our future.

Continue with the shoulders by crossing one arm in front of your chest, but keeping it straight, so it is essentially reaching in the other direction. Pull and reach with the arm, until you feel the stretch in the back of the shoulder blade. You can stretch the biceps by holding onto a wall with one hand, arm straight, and twist away with the rest of your body until you feel a stretch in the upper arm. To stretch the triceps, simply lift one arm and bend it at the elbow with the forearm reaching downward toward the middle of the upper back. Switch and make sure you do both arms. In a standing position, you can take advantage and stretch the quads, or upper thighs, by bending one knee with the foot pointing upward behind you until you feel the pull in the front part of the upper leg. Switch and do the other one too. To stretch the calves, you can lunge out with one leg forward, knee bent, and keep the other leg perfectly straight, with toes also pointing forward. Hold for a few moments until you feel a good stretch in the calf of the straight leg, then repeat with the other leg.

Stretching can be as simple or as elaborate as you need it to be. There are stretches that involve props, such as elastic bands, which are excellent for the less flexible among us, who need an extra hand to achieve the deeper stretch. Elastic bands are great because there are different levels of resistance, so you can experiment with what works for you, and you can always throw them in your bag to have on hand for any member of the family, anywhere you go.

Of course, there are all kinds of stretches you can do that require nothing but your sheer will to get through. An excellent lower back stretch and chest opener, for instance, is to simply lie on your belly with hands close to your shoulders and legs stretched back, held straight. Gently push your upper body upward, which lengthens and stretches the lower spine, and hold the posture for at least ten seconds, while breathing deeply.

To stretch the legs, stand with feet parallel and wide apart, and bend down on one knee, keeping the other leg straight. Take a few deep breaths there and switch sides. This can naturally move us along into a straddle, and everyone should open up his/her legs as wide as possible, to feel a good stretch but not a painful one. Make sure your kids can differentiate between the two. Sit up straight with hands in front of you, and slowly reach forward as far as you can, always remembering to push harder on the exhale, and making every push deliberate and gentle. Always keep in mind that it is crucial not just to get your kids to start stretching—it is just as key to make sure they are stretching *right*.

From the straddle position, reach with one arm over your head and stretch to one side, looking upward, and on the front side of your stretched arm. Try to touch your toes with your reaching arm, and feel the stretch all along one side of your upper body. Let the opposite arm glide across the floor, palm up, in the opposite direction. The more flexible ones among us can aim to touch the shoulder to the floor.

Continue to stretch the glutes by lying on your back and holding your knees up to a 90-degree angle, your hips level with your knees. Now cross one ankle over one knee, and reach with both arms through the opposite bent knee until you feel the stretch deeply in one of the buttocks. You can then sit up and stretch the outer thigh by crossing one leg over the other, with the knee bent and foot flat on the floor. Then simply twist in the opposite direction with the upper body until you feel it in the outer part of the upper leg. You can get a deep stretch in the hamstring by lying back down and raising one leg up toward your head, holding the leg with both hands at the calves for proper support and guidance.

Finally, lie on your back and bring both knees to your chest with your arms wrapped tightly around them, for a deep stretch in the lower back.

One of the great things about stretching is the fact that you can always pair up and assist each other for deeper impact. Sometimes, just the presence of another person there cheering you on, or spotting you for safety, is all you really need to get through the drills. Also, a stretching partner can help ease your muscles into the more challenging positions, and can help to remind you to breathe when you're moving in and out of the postures. For a very simple partnered hamstring stretch, one person can lie on the ground with both legs straight, while the other partner helps raise the leg, in a straight position, to a maximum stretch. The assisting partner can gradually help to move you into a more challenging expression of the stretch, while also making sure that you are safe as you move through it.

There are some other basic things you should also always keep in mind and impart to your family members when they're stretching.

- **Breathe deeply while you stretch to help your body move oxygen-rich blood to those sore muscles.**

- **When you stretch, ease your body gradually into the postures, until you feel a mild pull on your muscles, tendons, and ligaments. A stretch should never hurt.**

- Hold a stretch for 30 seconds or more. Wait 15 to 30 seconds before you stretch the next group of muscles.

- Don't bounce, and don't force yourself into an uncomfortable position.

- Stretch before and after exercise as part of your warm-up and cooling-down routine.

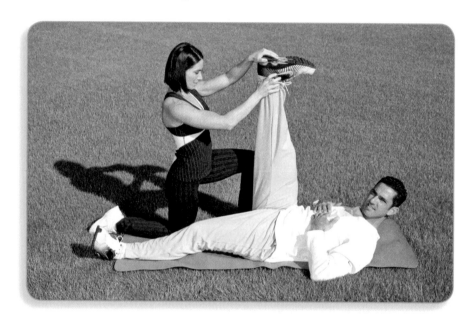

WORDS OF ENCOURAGEMENT

Not all kids are as naturally active as others, and many will take a little extra nudge to get the ball rolling, so to speak. Remember your role as motivator and hype man, but be crafty in your approach so it doesn't sound like nagging. The best way of motivating is by *being active yourself* and by providing positive feedback and support when your kids show an interest in being active. Encourage group lessons or teams if kids show a particular inclination in any direction, and if they don't, expose them to a wide array of things early on, so that they can start homing in on what they like most.

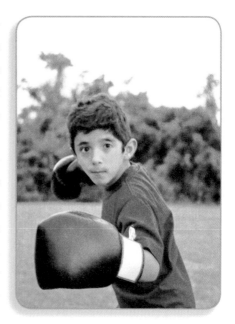

To encourage positivity with your kids, celebrate them with words of praise when they do well, rather than focusing on their negatives. Notice their progress and congratulate them for their successes. Help them understand and tap into that adrenaline-pumped feeling of being a winner.

Anytime your child wants to show you progress in an activity, receive it with all of your attention, and honor their efforts by responding with positive affirmations. In doing so, you will be consciously strengthening their self-esteem, allowing them to see that their hard work is worthy, and that progress and success are only as far away as they are willing to work for them. If your child can show unbridled confidence on a sporting field, you better believe they will likely show that same confidence in life.

The Reason's the Season

This section is meant to remind you that the universe is a perfect playground on which you can play out your new agenda of fun family fitness. It is meant to show everyone that the seasons are the most natural, built-in reasons to stay active, and that when acknowledged properly, they can forge a sense of connectedness to nature and all of the beautiful wonders that it brings, year-round.

There are so many reasons to use nature as your guide. First and foremost, it allows everyone to connect with their surroundings, and to feel and experience awareness and appreciation for the details, those stunning little blessings that we get in the form of magenta sunsets, giant snowflakes, leaves in vivid orange and red tones, and white foaming waves crashing in a perfect rage over a shell-speckled shore. All of those, and countless more, are there for us to enjoy—if we are smart enough to plan accordingly and *get outside*. Getting the family outside is like going back to basics in the most pure, wholesome, and therapeutic way. It reminds us of what life is all about and creates the building blocks of what will ultimately become our most long-lasting memories.

All you have to do is commit to planning a bit, provide all the right gear—such as proper clothes for rain or snow and all relevant safety equipment—and remain strong in your role as the motivator, organizer, and coordinator of the group.

THE SEASONAL BREAKDOWN

Needless to say, the notion of "seasons" is relative, as people live in all varieties of climates and regions, and so everyone's sense of season will tend to vary. That said, take the following breakdown with a grain of salt and adapt it to your own needs, depending on where you live and what *your* individual seasonal possibilities may offer. In Florida, for example, there are not really four distinct seasons, so a lot of the summer activities will be relevant to people who live there year-round. Families in Colorado and Utah, on the other hand, might relate more to the winter activities. You get the point. The main idea is to look closely at everything around you and commit to nurturing your family's connection to it. Also, keep in mind that many of the activities can overlap into other seasons. We listed trampoline, for example, under autumn, but if you have access to a trampoline in the summertime—by all means, get bouncing. We simply itemized them this way to give you a wide array of ideas to have at your fingertips for each season. Get creative and be flexible, especially when it comes to the outdoor activities that can easily be done in the summer, spring, or fall.

Remember above all that fitness should not have to be thought of as a cost and should not, under any circumstances, end up under the domain of annoying burdens in your life. Before you start making excuses about how exercising is too expensive, do research in your area about special programs for families at gyms and family centers that may offer reduced costs, family packages, or free courses. Certain facilities have discounts on certain days, so if you get resourceful and dive into the information that is out there for you, your family won't ever miss a beat. Also, keep in mind that many gyms today have day care services now, so you can get your workout even if you're a brand-new mom with a busy schedule. Check into swim nights at a middle school or high school pool; YMCA; community center classes and sports; Mommy and Me; and even libraries.

Spring

The Season of Possibility

There is nothing quite like the enchantment of spring, that magical time of newness, of fresh possibilities and the aroma of blooming buds swirling together in the crisp air. In this season, the grass boasts its greenest green, the birds sing with more chirpy gusto, the flowers open up in a proud display, and the colors of everything pop in crisp synchronicity. Spring is nature at her most glorious, ripe, and robust, and for that reason, it is one of the best times of the year to be outside.

We happen to love spending our springs visiting orchards and farms where we can pick fruits like fresh strawberries and spend entire days under a perfect blue sky, fully connected to the earth around us. And because the weather is so pleasant this time of the year, we try to play as many sports outside as possible. Be it in a park or in our own backyard, we don't miss a beat when it comes to spring.

Gardening

The magic of gardening with your children becomes evident on so many levels: they understand and connect with the universe just by digging their little hands into the earth; they see and feel where their food comes from and in this way gain awareness that they will surely carry forward. Gardening is one of those activities that engages the upper body, especially the back and arms, and it's so much fun, you don't even realize you are working out by digging, planting, picking, and pruning. Gardening is active, universal, essential, and ultimately deeply fulfilling, and sharing this activity as a family, where the group can reap the results together, is always a special experience. Try to plant things that you know you will later use in your kitchen. For example, we love to grow herbs such as basil, thyme, rosemary, and mint. Try it and enjoy the full-circle experience of utilizing what you grow yourself.

Tree Climbing

When we were growing up we often visited our grandparents at their house in the mountains, where there were many amazing trees. All of the cousins would climb those trees as a matter of ritual. We would all climb up into the entanglement of branches and stay up there talking for hours. The little ones, of course, couldn't always get up there, and I remember being up there and looking down at the poor souls who didn't make it up. Being up in the tree gave you status; it meant you were in the club, you were cool. Climbing trees is a universal classic, and it is the kind of thing that can really stamp our childhoods

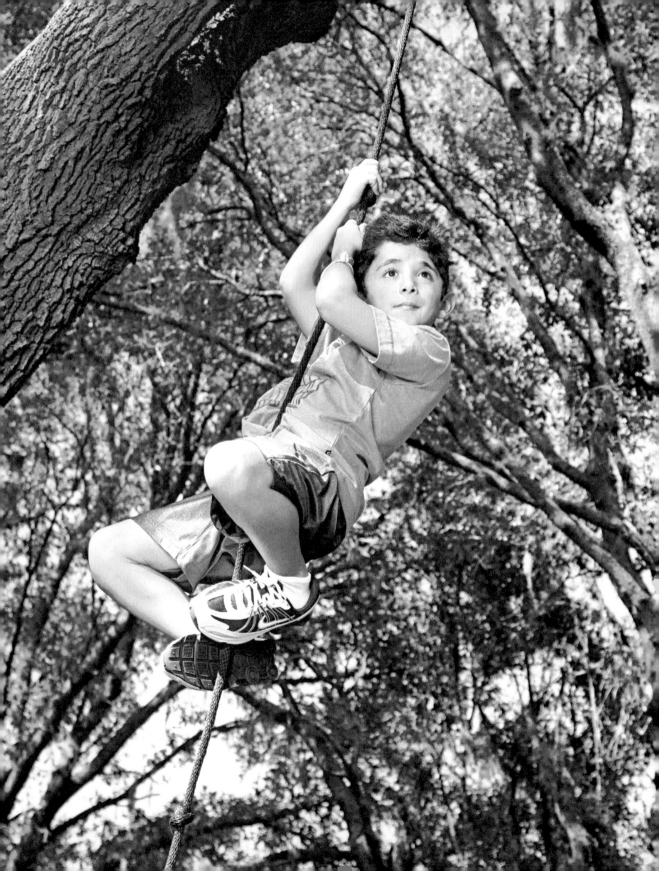

with unforgettable memories. Rule number one is to loosen up and trust that your child will not actually attempt something that is too dangerous for him or her. More important is to watch them and be there as a spot, just in case. We love letting our kids play and climb on trees because it encourages a sense of pioneering and confidence and gets them to connect with nature, bark-to-hands.

Tennis

Tennis, anyone? We say, *Tennis, everyone!* Tennis is not only a tremendously thorough form of exercise but also carries with it a sense of tradition, elegance, and gracefulness. It introduces your children to an activity that is at once competitive and quite refined. Tennis is also nice because it can be both solitary and collaborative, depending on whether you are playing singles or doubles. Tennis is a game you can learn early in life and practice at any age. It is a sport that binds the generations, and for that reason invites everyone in the family to participate. If you don't know how to play the game, you can also take classes along with your kids, showing them that it is never too late to learn.

Soccer

Considering that there is a global obsession with soccer, even if you live within the culture of soccer, as a parent you are essentially educating your children about world recreation when you introduce them to soccer early in their lives. Don't feel that you have to have two whole teams in place to play; by simply running the ball, practicing footwork, and blocking goals, your kids will start to understand and appreciate the elements of the game.

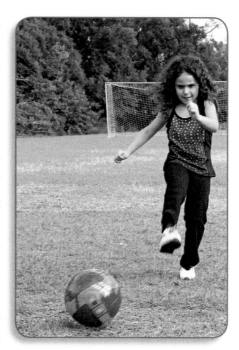

Dodgeball

We always played dodgeball in school. If your kids have the backbone for it, playing dodgeball is an exercise in developing fortitude. It teaches kids to stand with courage, move defensively, and stay alert, all in the spirit of playful aggression. It's OK to get fierce and feisty—after all, won't those traits come in handy later on in life? Just make sure, however, that you set ground rules about how hard they can throw—especially if you have boys playing with girls.

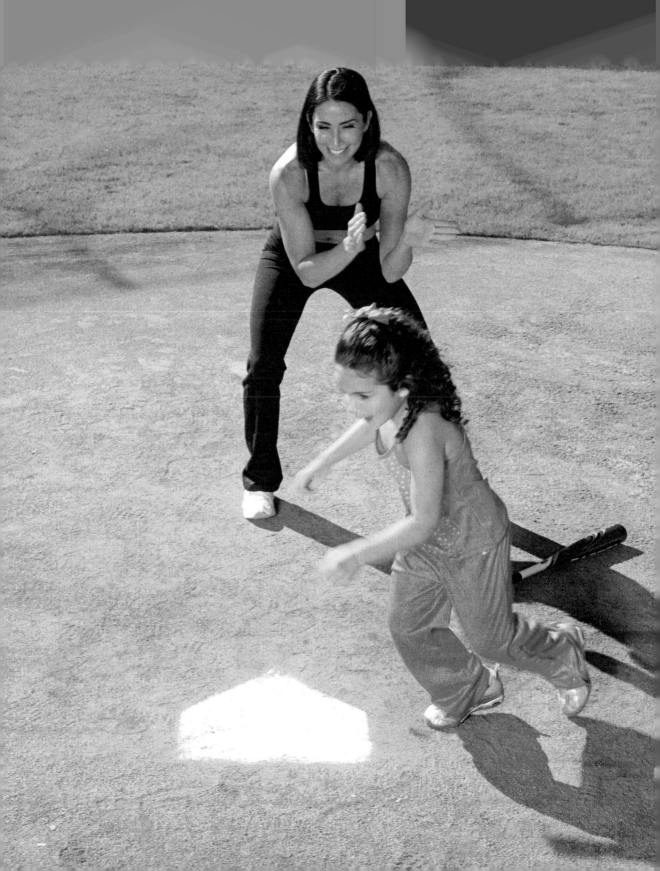

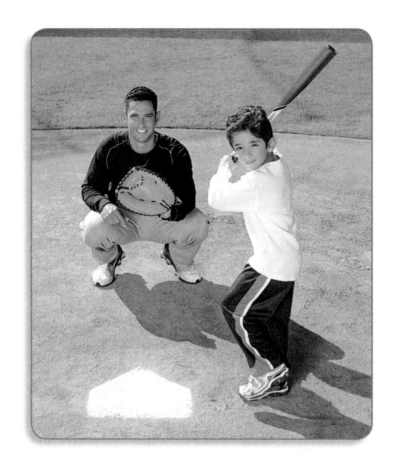

Baseball

In the spirit of the apple falling not far from the tree, as Posadas, baseball is something of a life force for us—so, of course, whenever we get a chance to play as a family, even if it's just the four of us, it is an absolute joy. It doesn't matter if you don't have enough players, as the game can be simply about practicing pitching, catching, and running the bases. This way, the kids don't have a chance to get bored—they can keep switching from catcher to pitcher, which keeps the activities dynamic, fluid, and fun.

Basketball

Basketball has always been one of our favorites because of how consistently active it is. It helps kids understand the importance of staying on their toes, of being vigilant and quick, and of collaborating and synchronizing with other players. The little ones can simply dribble the ball, and you'll see that that alone can be endlessly thrilling to them, what with the rhythm of the ball against the ground and the notion that they themselves can control it, each child gradually working on their own personal missions of one day sinking a basket or blocking a shot.

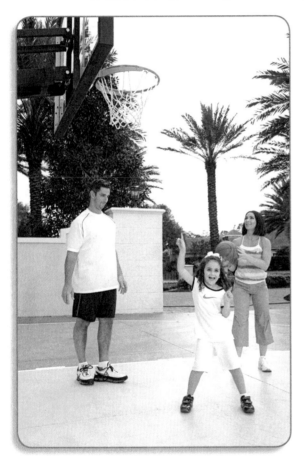

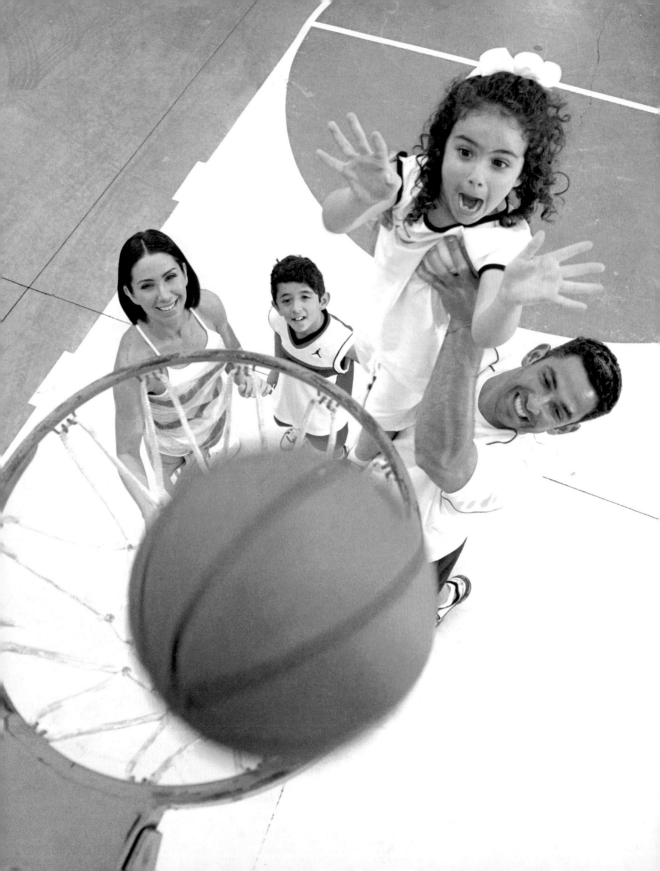

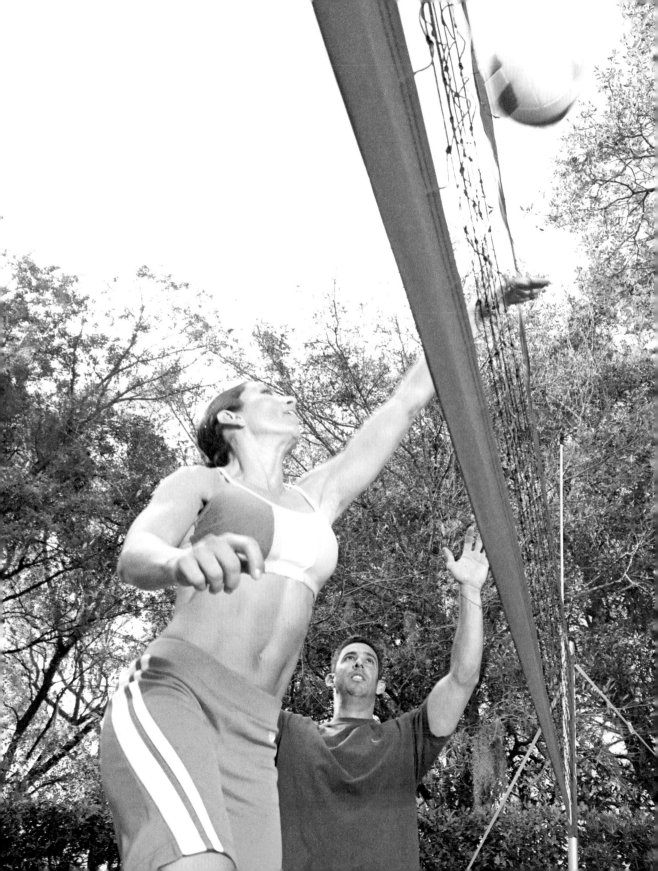

Volleyball

We grew up playing volleyball, so we definitely have a soft spot for it. If it seems like it is too rough on the arms of small children, you might want to start with a simplified version of the game, called Newcomb, where instead of hitting the ball with the undersides of their arms, the kids catch the ball and then throw it back and forth over the net. Don't get us wrong, if they're up to the challenge of volleying, don't hold them back. You can also practice with a lighter beach ball in the pool. From our experience, kids love volleyball. Our daughter, Paulina, is six years old and she cannot get enough of it. All you need is a ball, two people, and a couple of drills, and everyone has a great time.

Kickball

We know it may sound crazy, but if you want to be thorough about your children's fitness, think anatomically. As you brainstorm your programs and activities, try to ensure that *all* of their little parts get worked out—which is why we *adore* kickball. As they run after the ball and learn how to kick with all their might, the kids develop their leg muscles and stamina, and certainly become poised to play soccer, and countless other sports, later on. You can practice basic drills, or you can make a weekend of it and conduct full-scale kickball tournaments with teams comprised of friends or relatives. Kickball is also great because the rules of the game are similar to those of baseball, so it also has the power to get kids thinking about that sport down the line.

Skateboarding

The skateboard is another one of those "letting go" activities that is absolutely thrilling to many children. Provided everyone is wearing the right protective gear, the skateboard encourages kids to trust themselves, find balance, and really go for it. Even just starting out basically, by exploring how to move on a skateboard, can be fun—and has the added benefit, by virtue of the kinds of movements required, of also preparing them for snowboarding and surfing when they're older. If your kids seem to be into it, check out local skateboarding parks for children, and look into getting them some lessons.

Miniature Golf

Miniature golf is a perfect Saturday or Sunday kind of plan that puts everyone in a good mood. It's the perfect balance of sportsmanship and whimsy, the kind of activity that makes for excellent family quality time. Even the grandparents can join in, and we know our parents enjoy it just as much as our kids do every time we do it as a family. It is wonderful because it puts everyone on the same playing level. Most cities have a local miniature golf court of some kind, so do some research, and surprise your kids one day. You will not regret it.

Summer

The Season of Jubilation

Summertime . . . and the living *is* easy. There is nothing like summertime to get everyone's juices flowing, with that special warm and balmy air on our sun-kissed skin, and the freedom of not having to wear eight million layers. Summer, to us, is the smell of a fresh watermelon, homemade lemonade, and anything with coconut in it. Summer is the beach, the pool, and a backyard BBQ, when days feel endless and time seems to stand still. Summer is the sound of seagulls and the smell of salty sea air; it is the season of long, lingering afternoons, where the notion of pure leisure can be fully experienced and expressed. Use your summers wisely, as your kids will have large chunks of free time. Make the most of it by always having activities laid out as options, and of course never let up on the sunscreen during the hot summer months.

Swimming

Swimming is one of those activities that stays with your children forever. This one is sacred. Be it the ocean, a local lake, or a pool in the summertime, there is no getting around the fact that swimming makes for good old-fashioned fun. Not to mention the fact that swimming is also one of the most physically comprehensive activities for optimal physical fitness. We are firm believers that teaching your children how to swim—and, more important, teaching them how to *enjoy* swimming—is one of the most invaluable lessons you can give them. Remember that with swimming, particularly in the ocean, there comes a whole array of other activities, such as snorkeling, which our daughter is crazy about, waterskiing, and jet-skiing.

We would be remiss if we did not reemphasize here the importance of safety when it comes to swimming. First of all, it is never too early to teach your kids to swim, and you should think of teaching them this critical skill set as a matter of safety first and foremost. And even when they do know how to swim, adults should *always* be present *and watching* when kids are in the pool, and certainly in the ocean. We've heard too many horror stories about accidents at pool parties, so we are hard-core advocates of parents seriously monitoring pool or ocean time.

Beach

Introducing your children to the beach when they are babies is the equivalent of handing them a little slice of heaven to

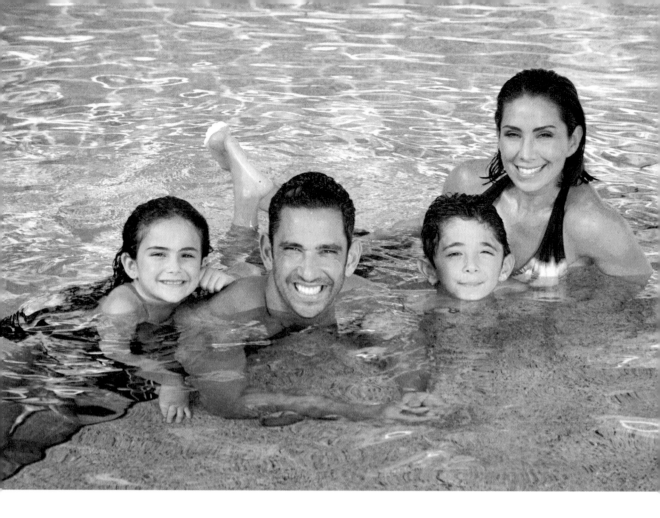

carry around for the rest of their lives. Family beach outings are wonderfully versatile as far as activities go—because you can play everything from catch, tag, volleyball, and paddleball, to sand castle competitions, swimming, or simply taking nice long walks along the shore. As long as everyone is properly geared up with ample sunscreen, you can think of the beach as the ideal setting in which to carry out any number of different plans—a place where tranquility and appreciation for nature and fun meet right in the palms of your kids' little hands.

When we went to the beach as kids with our father, he would meticulously explain to us about the movement of the waves and how to navigate in those waves. He taught us when to go under and how to catch a wave so that we could be carried safely to shore. He taught us never to turn our back on the ocean, and always to show it our utmost respect. Remember to teach your children about the power and magnitude of the ocean.

—*Laura Posada*

Sand Sculptures

When you're lying around at the beach, *don't just lie there*. Always aim to be active and engaged. If you don't feel like playing a game or running around too much, why not work on a sand sculpture? You can work on one giant sculpture as a group, like a giant mermaid, using shells for her bra and seaweed for her hair; or each one can work on their own project and make a competition out of it. The point is that the beach is full of natural accessories and treasures with which to enhance your sculptures, so that you can really milk the natural inspiration that can come from a perfect day at the beach. Bring buckets of different sizes and shovels so you can mold and detail in different ways. You can also use the buckets to collect seaside accoutrements to bring all your sculptures to life.

Paddleball

We grew up playing paddleball on the perfect beaches of Puerto Rico; in fact, there was no such thing as a beach outing without a set of paddles and the little rubber ball. Later, as adults, when we were traveling in Israel visiting some friends, we were delighted and surprised to see the prevalence of paddleball on the beaches of Tel Aviv. That showed us how universally loved and practiced the game really is! The metric sound of the small black rubber ball gives the game a rhythmic, cadenced character, which is immensely calming and therapeutic on a hot summer beach day—and the game has the added benefit of being a total body workout. Best of all, the paddles and balls are portable enough to keep in your beach bag always.

Slip 'N Slide

My children would begin every morning of their lives on a Slip 'n Slide if they could. They go absolutely crazy for it, and frankly, so do we. Slip 'n Slide is a summertime staple that makes everyone happy because it is refreshing, adventurous, a full-body activity, and endlessly entertaining to do and watch. If you want to see your children laughing hysterically and high on life, get them a Slip 'n Slide. If you *really* want to make them laugh, hurl across the thing yourself! If we can do it, you can do it.

Pool

It is no mystery that kids love pools, and when you open your mind about activities that are possible in the pool, you can help take their experience to the next level. Water aerobics, for example, can be really fun and fulfilling for restless little ones who want a physical challenge when they are splashing around. You can even conduct treading water competitions (ages and abilities pending), to see who can hold out the longest, an excellent way to work on leg strength and stamina. Even good old Marco Polo works in the pool—anything that keeps the group active, focused, and happy. Our kids love to play a pool game called torpedoes, which is basically nothing more than throwing objects to the bottom of the pool and having races to see who can swim down and retrieve them first. There are all kinds of variations, like who can gather the most items, or who can gather them first, and so on. Get creative, and make sure to keep a close eye on the kids when they are playing this one.

Car Washing

On a hot summer day, a group car wash can be deliciously refreshing, and also productive, which we *love*. But don't just wash the car—make an event out of it: whip up a batch of fresh lemonade, bring out a boom box, and have some fun. This one is smart because it demonstrates the power of group effort, and the sense that chores can actually be a good time, if you have the right attitude about them. All of that, and the car will actually be clean again by the end of the day—what can beat that?

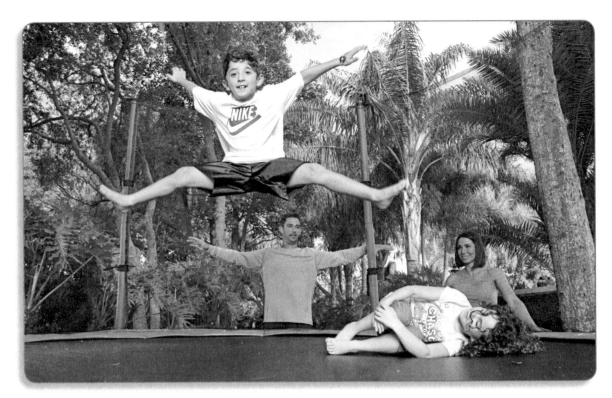

Trampoline

This is an all-time favorite in our house. The magic of the trampoline is that it allows the kids to adventurously explore their sense of gravity and balance while also helping to hone and develop their acrobatic skills. The trampoline is phenomenal because in addition to its physical benefits, it also works on your kids' sense of courage and their ability to "let go." After all, it can be tremendously liberating to fly up in the air like that, knowing that you are safe . . . especially when you are a child.

A note about safety here: you should always have a safety net, and you should be especially watchful of big kids jumping with little kids, because they are jumping at very different levels, and it could get too intense for the smaller ones. Also be very careful of flips, because unless someone actually knows what they are doing, they can break their neck.

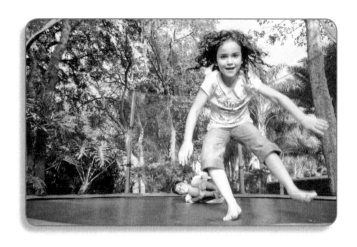

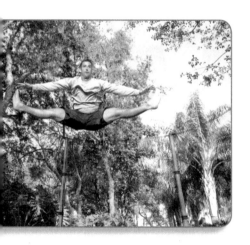

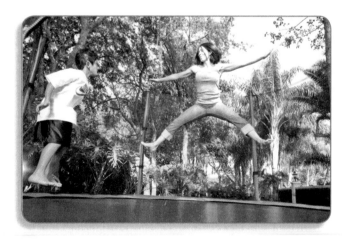

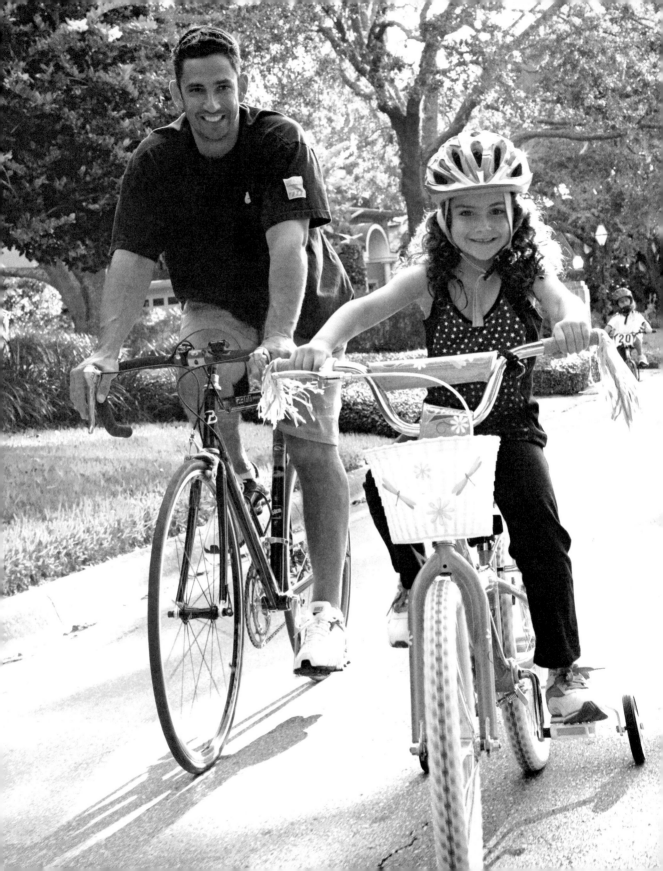

Bicycling

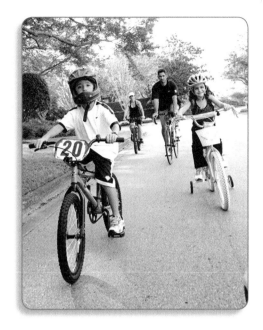

There is nothing like gearing up the whole clan on a crisp, sunlit day and collectively chartering a course on bikes. We know, as parents of two young children, that we feel so complete somehow when we go out on a bike ride as a group, the wind in our faces, and the scenic routes that we get to share and enjoy. We strongly believe that as a general rule, if you can bike it, bike it. Ride the bikes to school, to the park, wherever. It's good exercise, and it's the environmental way to travel. Nothing wrong with going green while you go lean, right?

Biking is also a great thing to do when you travel—there's no better way to see a city than from the seat of your bicycle. There are all kinds of bike tours that cities offer, so look into it, and offer your family a new perspective on the art of travel. At home, there are community biking teams that get together on a weekly or biweekly basis and charter all kinds of amazing excursions. Check your local bike shops for this kind of information.

The way we see it, a bike ride is more than just a bike ride—it is a comprehensive physical activity that works the core, lower body, and heart; it places your family directly in touch with their surroundings, with nature, with the world. It is a dynamic, active journey, and most fun when you experience it with the people you love.

Autumn

The Season of Change

Autumn, or fall, is the season of total transformation. It is a time of return and renewal, when the universe seems to be on the brink of something epic—a season both blatantly stunning and delightfully melancholic. Autumn is a fantastic time, given the pleasant, not-too-hot temperatures and the explosive displays of red, yellow, and orange. For those lucky enough to live in areas where the foliage changes, we encourage you to embrace this piece of good fortune and get creative about what kinds of activities you can do against the backdrop of this special natural beauty.

Apple and Pumpkin Picking

You can of course garden with your kids at home—but you can take it to the next level by bringing them on fruit and vegetable picking expeditions to farms, where they can pick and taste seasonal produce and participate, hands-on, in the process of the harvest. We never miss a chance to get out to the orchards and vineyards, and for our family, the feeling of coming home with our own handpicked goods is unparalleled. We truly

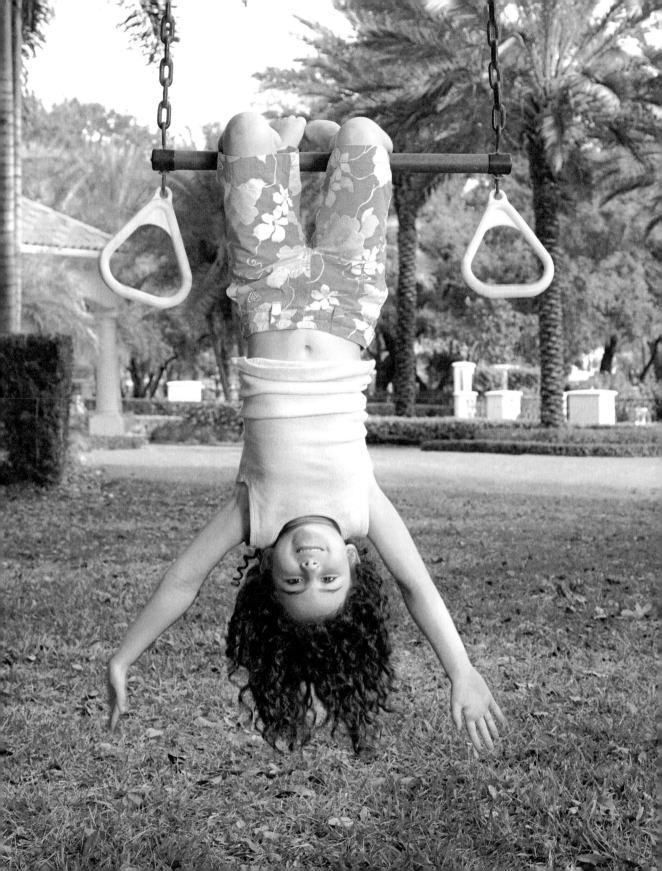

believe these types of earth-related activities have the power to impart a special sense of appreciation and connectedness to your kids.

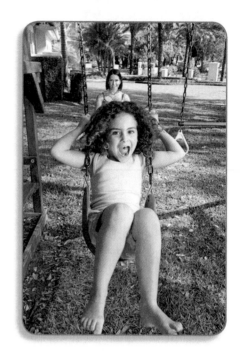

Wheelbarrows— *(Carretilla)*

This one is just plain goofy—and that's *exactly* why you should do it. Everyone involved laughs, and everyone gets an excellent arm workout. You don't need anything but yourselves and a little pep to get started. You can't go wrong. Have the kids do races, and just make sure they all switch positions (from wheelbarrow driver to wheelbarrow rider, and vice versa), so everyone gets the full challenge. These are fun to do in the fall when the ground is covered with beautiful autumn leaves.

Playground

It is time to rethink your idea of what a playground is. Gone should be the notion that a playground is a place for you to drop off your kids so that you can pal around, cappuccino in hand, with the moms on the sidelines; instead, think of the playground as a mini-gym for your kids, and *you* as their God-given trainer. Get right in there with them; we promise it will reinvigorate your sense of youth. Give them tasks (age and ability pending), such as crossing the monkey bars, hanging

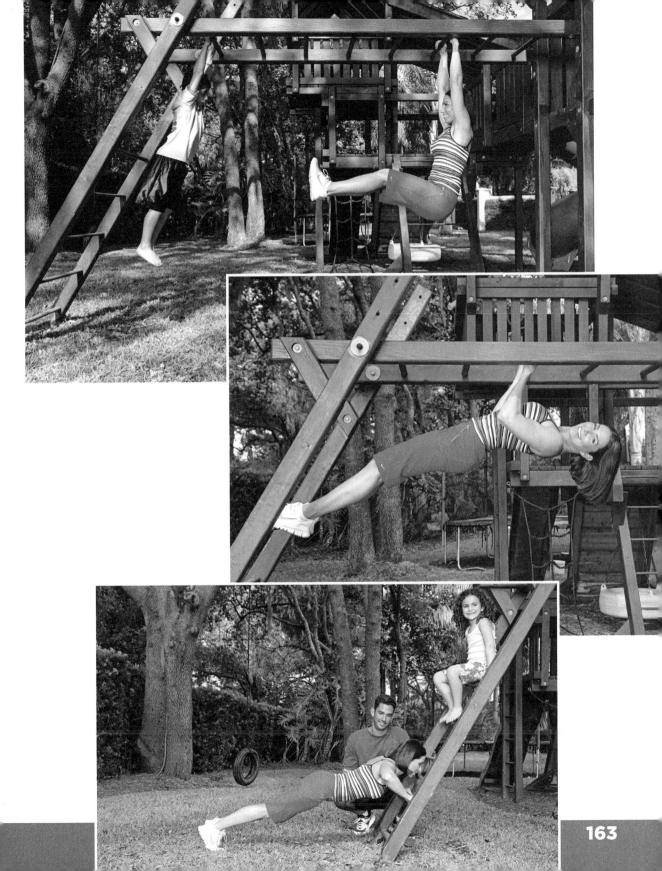

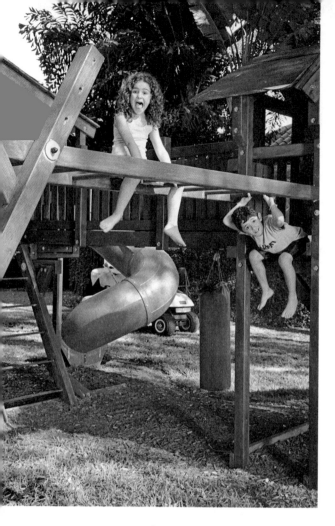

from their arms; doing chin-ups there; or walking upward on the slide, against gravity. Get creative about each day's agenda, so that the playground becomes a place of endless possibilities for them.

Boot Camp

Boot camp is always a favorite in our house because our kids love the sense of challenge and competition. The fun part about this one is that you can really ham up the drama and get serious with them. Get yourself a whistle and play the part of drill sergeant, all in good, playful fun. Time their tasks, and challenge them each time to try to break their own records. Keep logs of their progress, so they have a tangible way of seeing and measuring their own success. Get them excited about this process. Needless to say, you know your own kids and how much they'll be able to endure—but you will find, as we have, that children can really get into the idea of pushing their limits. It fuels them with drive and motivation and makes them feel grown-up and serious about play.

Boxing and Kickboxing

Don't be afraid to let your kids and spouses tap into their inner Rocky, as boxing and kickboxing both demand the integration of powerful limbs, balance, and determination to practice simple drills. These exercises, such as uppercuts, simple sparring, and strong leg kicks, can be especially exciting, fueling one with a sense of power and invincibility, and all at once giving excellent tone to the muscles. In our house, when the gloves come on, it's showtime.

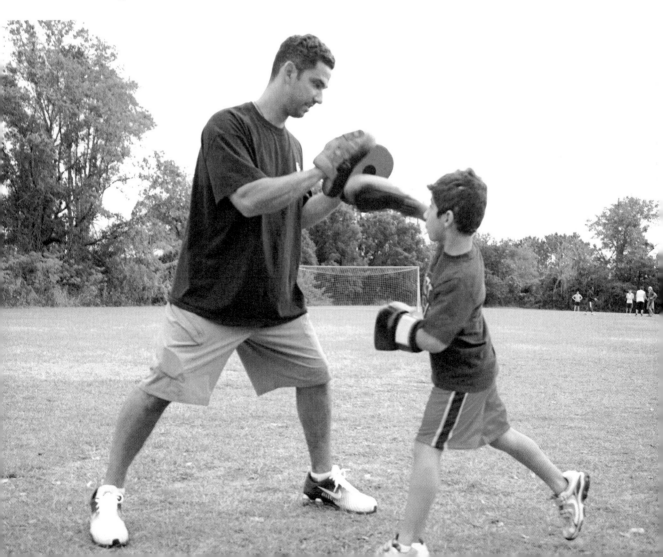

Flying Disk

Our kids love this one, and so do we. The soft flying disk is part Frisbee, part kite flying, and it is perfectly safe for kids of all ages to play. It's the next level of catch. This one is great because it is so incredibly simple but works simultaneously on aim, precision, direction, and collaboration. We love the flying disk because it is four times as large as a Frisbee, and therefore stays in the air for an extended period of time, which gives the little ones more of a chance to play and participate. It's also a lot less hard, and therefore safer than, say, a Frisbee, for small children. We use it to play monkey in the middle, which always turns out to be a crowd-pleaser.

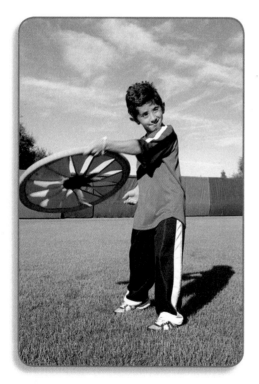 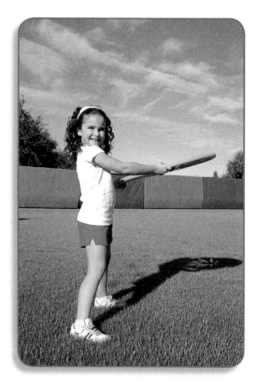

Winter

The Season of Inner Warmth

We didn't have winters as kids in Puerto Rico; now that we do, we milk as many opportunities as possible to maximize them. We remember seeing snow for the first time when we were sixteen, and totally freaking out about it as some kind of natural miracle. *It is!* So, if you live in a place where it snows, get out there and enjoy it. Enjoy the marvel of the whole thing, and be grateful that you, unlike a lot of other people, get to touch it with your very own hands. Remember that winter is all about cozying up to your own warmth and turning inward, a time of reflection and inner heat.

Skiing and Snowboarding

If you live anywhere near the right topography and climate, it is pretty much your duty to introduce skiing and/or snowboarding to your kids. This idea is also great if you are trying to come up with a unique family vacation—one where everyone can be active and on. Snow sports expose children to an entirely different dimension of exercise and fitness and show them an aspect of nature that you can be certain they will appreciate. If you're not sure whether to go with skiing *or* snowboarding, let your kids try both, and ask which appeals to them more. Usually a person feels more comfortable with one or the other, but the nice part of the plan is that skiers and snowboarders can all enjoy the same slopes. Maybe Mom and Sis ski, and Dad and the sons snowboard. Or vice versa! The point is that everyone can be together. There are facilities that offer reduced rates on certain days, or special family packages, so don't let the high cost of this activity scare you and your family from being able to do it. For those who don't enjoy downhill skiing, there is cross-country, which provides an incredible workout.

Sledding

In Puerto Rico we didn't have snow, but that certainly did not stop us from sledding down the steep grassy knoll located on the fort in the old city of San Juan. We would throw ourselves down that slope full force, gliding down to the base of the hill with all of the freedom in the world. Sledding is a fully liberating activity that allows one to fully surrender—and also involves the climb back up the hill for the next run down. Make sure everyone is wearing protective gear, especially helmets, but get creative about what everyone can sled on. Garbage can lids work wonders!

Snowshoeing

If the snow is deep enough, snowshoeing is fun, if not funny. Strapped onto one's feet, those awkward, giant snowshoes work the legs in a comprehensive way and keep everyone cracking up in the process!

Ice-skating

We recommend you learn ice-skating early, when it doesn't hurt so much to fall on the ice, and when you are less afraid of such a fall. Kids are somehow freer on the ice, so take advantage of that, and expose them to it early. We say it from experience, because when we go ice-skating with our children, we are the ones who are scared and they are the ones cheering us on, which is a nice change. They can motivate you as much as you can motivate them. Don't worry about genders here, because both can have fun on the ice. Boys may be inclined to play ice hockey as they get older, in which case ice-skating is something they will need to have mastered. Girls, on the other hand, might be inclined to practice figure skating. Either way, getting kids on ice early in life offers them more possibilities, and as they get older they will be more empowered to be selective about the hobbies and activities they choose for themselves. Also, ice-skating instills a sense of confidence, as well as poise.

Snowball Fights

When a fresh snow comes down and graces us with its vast white beauty, there is nothing more fun then engaging in an all-out, no-holds-barred snowball battle with the closest members of your family. Snowball fights, while endlessly mischievous and totally wild, also encourage arm strength, endurance, personal determination, and courage—so get on out into the fresh snow and declare snowball war!

Building Snowmen

Again, if you are lucky enough to get a weekend full of fresh snow, one of the most fun things you can do as a group is to build snow people. Build entire families of them, and really get creative. Make all kinds of funny tableau situations, and really have fun with how you accessorize your frosty friends. This gets all kinds of artful juices flowing but also works the arms and back with all of the digging and patting down of snow.

Snow Angels

This is an old favorite that never bores. Kids love it, and we cannot deny it, adults do just as much. There is nothing like throwing yourself, belly up, into a pile of fresh powder and flapping your extremities with abandon to create perfect angels of snow. Snow angels are little morsels of nostalgia; they are one of those ever-sweet bites of life that stay with you always and make you want to teach them to your kids.

The Triple A's

Anytime, Anywhere Activities

There is of course a whole world of other types of activities that you can do anywhere, anytime—the kinds of games that can just spring up, off-the-cuff, impromptu, and sometimes these very moments of total spontaneity are the most fun. These are activities and games that you can take with you on the road, on your family vacations, to the grandparents' house, *anywhere*. All they really require is the will to participate, as they are universal in their approach, ease, and appeal.

Core Strength

There is no getting around it: core strength represents solid structural integrity. It is the base of all our power, and if we are taught this basic tenet of proper fitness early in our lives, we become prepared to have strong bellies in the future. For some reason, we don't start getting serious about our abdominal workouts until it is too late and our belly rolls abound. But the most basic, logical thing is to start getting kids motivated to work on their core strength as early as possible. Do your abs

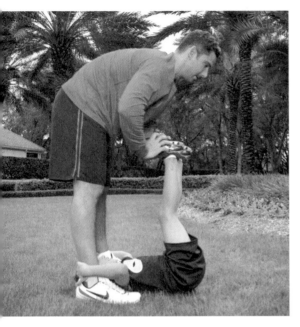

exercises not only for your abs to be tight—do them so that your kids will see you doing them, and hopefully be inspired to do the same. Start with basic crunches, with arms bent behind the head, hands holding the head, knees bent, and feet flat on the floor; you can then try variations, pointing both knees in one direction and doing the crunches that way, to develop and work on your oblique muscles. Now try a set of crunches with both legs in the air, to strengthen your lower belly, which tends to be a tricky area to manage.

If you think sit-ups and crunches are the only way to achieve strong and sturdy abs, we dare you to take it up a notch by working in some new and dynamic abdominal exercises, which are easy, collaborative, and effective if done regularly. Here's one that we love: get into teams of partners—father and son, or daughter and mom, for example. One of you lie on your

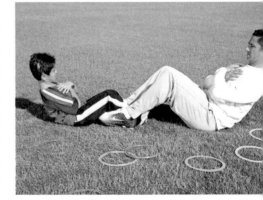

back with legs stretched upward and knees straight, reaching back with the arms to grip the ankles of the standing partner, who should stand right behind the top of the supine partner's head. The standing person should gently throw the legs of the supine person downward, while the person who is lying down uses his/

her own core strength and resistance to keep his/her legs up and straight. Do as many reps as you can, and whatever your individual records are, try to beat them every time by adding one or two more reps to each set, to gradually create more strength in your core.

Myachi

If you haven't hopped on the Myachi wave, now is the time. This small sand-filled hand sack is tossed around using the back of the hand. Any surface of the body can be used except the palm of the hand—and the whole point is not to let the sack hit the ground. It is a whole-body effort like no other; it asks you to engage your whole self, so it's a great workout, and best of all, the sack is small and portable enough to take anywhere and use anytime. Our kids go absolutely crazy for it.

Monkey in the Middle

All you need is a ball (or pillow, or stuffed toy, or water balloons . . . get creative) and three players for this one, and it is one you can essentially do anywhere. It's engaging and simple, and kids of all ages can easily play. Take this one to the beach, to the park, to the playground—and never be afraid to ignite a full-on, arms-up, smiles-wide monkey session with your kids.

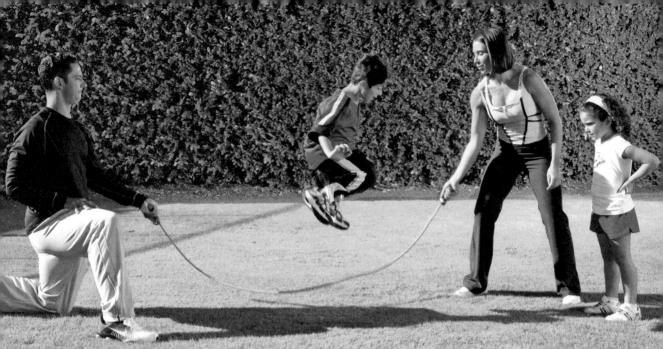

Jumping Rope

Jumping rope is one-stop shopping: it combines mastery of rhythm, stamina, endurance, and balance—and it can be done anywhere, from morning to night. Jumping rope is one of those things you can do alone or as a group, and a jump rope is so easy and light, you can just throw it in your bag, take it on a trip, or carry it around wherever you like. Best yet, it's one of the best cardiovascular workouts you can do. Think Rocky Balboa.

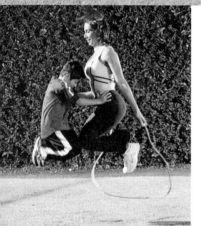

Tug-of-war

We always do an en masse family tug-of-war when we get together, and we take our victories and defeats very seriously indeed. The great tug-of-war puts "the team" into action like nothing else does, as every muscle, every stance, and every grip of every team member works in unison to achieve the goal of the group tug. It is so old school but so endlessly fun.

Medicine Balls and Balance Balls

Don't ask us why, but kids LOVE the balance ball. They want to sit on it, they want to throw it, they want to bounce on it. They just want it. It's like a magnet for kids; they should call it the *magnet ball*. The balance ball is great because it is an ideal indoor activity. Worked with properly, it can help promote flexibility, balance, strength, and coordination. The cool thing about this activity is that the balance ball is the kind of thing you can have anywhere in the house, always around, should someone feel the need to do a quick stretch session. Medicine balls are kind of like the weighted basketballs used frequently in physical therapy and sports rehabilitation. You can use them as extra weight for simple exercises, such as lunges and squats, and enchant your kids by explaining to them that even back in the days of ancient

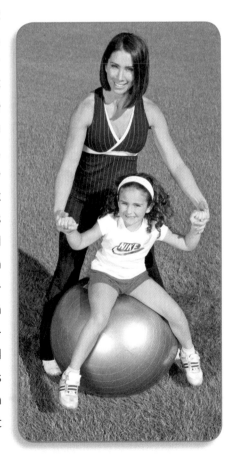

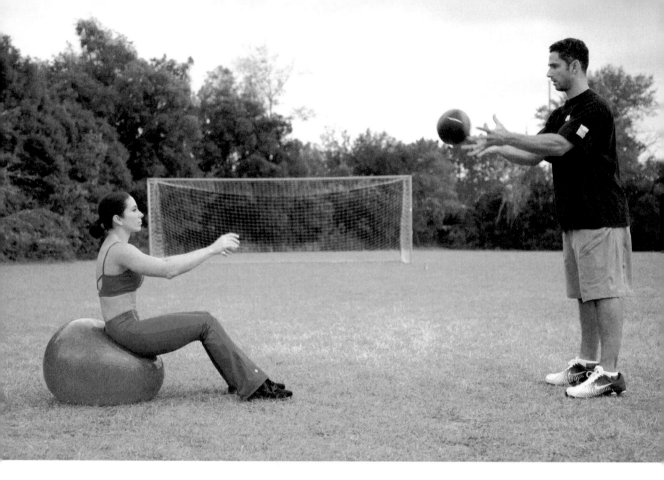

Greece, men used to throw and catch handmade sandbags, similar to medicine balls, at one another as a way to promote physical fitness. Make them feel like little warriors in their own right!

Hopscotch

This old favorite never bores. For some reason, throughout generations, kids have always adored hopscotch. When we introduced it to our daughter, she went nuts for it. We were surprised she didn't know about it, and were shocked when her little eyes lit up. What can you do? In our modern world, some of the old favorites can get lost. Think of yourselves as revitalizers, and bring back the old favorites by exposing your kids to them. Part of the fun of the

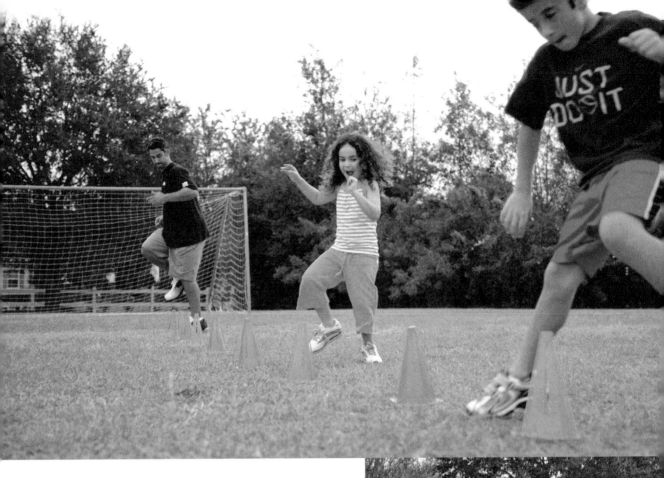

game is simply to bring the chalk out onto the street or sidewalk, and everyone can have some fun with outdoor chalk drawing. An ordinary game of hopscotch can turn into a butterfly-drawing competition just like that!

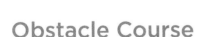

Obstacle Course

This one is fantastic for kids who are lazy or have short attention spans. It works on their ability to stay on task and also gets them off their bums. The obstacle course works indoors or outdoors, and much like a scavenger hunt, can be anything you want it to be. It's up to you to set something up that is entertaining, challenging, interactive, clever, and of course safe. Come up with obstacles that you know speak to things your kids love to do; keep them guessing, and enjoy watching them charge forward. Try things like relay races and use other running tasks that include the kids having to trade an object for another object; maybe set up little "pit stops" where they have to stop and do a set of sit-ups or a little dance. Have fun with it! Don't be afraid to mix physical challenges with more mental and even creative ones. Engage them with fun prizes, and exercise your own creativity to come up with the kind of game that will keep your kids remembering that day forever.

Walking

We don't think it's a coincidence that New Yorkers are known to have some of the longest life expectancies, considering how much walking they do every day. Walking is one of those activities that many people may forget or even take for granted simply because it is something we do (and have to do) to get around. But when you, as a family, go out for a long walk—a conscious, intentional walk, be it somewhere local or elsewhere—you essentially remind your children about the God-given basics of being human and impart the idea that there is never really an excuse for not getting up and moving your body—you can do it just by walking. It reminds them to go back to simple things, to appreciate every little step they take. Just like the rule about biking, the same applies here: when you can walk it, walk it, as this is one of the most basic ways you can get your body to move.

Tag

Sometimes the simplest things are the ones that make the most sense. Tag is one such phenomenon. We believe tag is genius because it can happen pretty much anywhere and it does not require any gear or equipment. Tag can be a tremendous workout. Chase someone for fifteen minutes and see how fast your heart rate shoots up. It is an old classic that is always relevant and also happens to be a fantastic cardiovascular workout for everyone. Believe it or not, our kids like to go to a tag class on Sundays; silly as it sounds, if it gets them running around with their friends for half an hour, we're happy.

INDOOR ACTIVITIES

We know we glorified nature earlier in the chapter and practically made you swear to do everything outside. And we still think you should! But sometimes, we know, it is simply not possible. Sometimes it's just too cold, or it's raining cats and dogs, or you all unanimously feel like having a late Sunday brunch and just doing stuff at home in your pajamas. Totally valid. We cannot and will not argue with that. Instead, we thought it would be productive to go over an array of *indoor* activities—the kind that you can bust out on a school night, on the weekends, day or night, all in the comfort of your own home. But don't just think of these as "indoor" activities; instead, see them as the kinds of things you can do with kids who don't love the notion of exercise or who aren't crazy about playing outside. Again, it is that subtle art of gently pushing your children into *doing,* by asking them to *do* things that are fun and perhaps slightly different than what they are used to.

Remember, your job is to be the instigator, the hype man, the motivator, and the planner. Step up to that challenge yourself, as a parent, and watch as your household evolves into a place of action and vitality.

Bowling

Bowling is the perfect answer to a rainy day. It's a step-out-of-the-box activity that is always a crowd-pleaser. You can team up and play parents against kids, or boys against girls. You can really jack up the significance of the whole thing by holding a faux tournament that carries on through the whole year or through the winter.

Yoga

For all those parents out there who believe yoga should be relegated to new age hippies or aging hipsters, its time to wake up and smell the incense, because yoga, believe it or not, is relevant to the ancient gurus of India, to hippies and hipsters, to you, *and* to your kids. Yoga is universal, and it will work on every element of your child's person: the mental, the physical, the emotional, and the spiritual. It will calm them, center them, and open their minds to a world of active tranquility. If nothing else, yoga will teach your child the importance of breath and the beauty of strong determination balanced with grace. If cost is an issue for you, and yoga classes are out of the question, get your hands on a DVD, such as *Yoga for Kids* (which we own and love) and practice with your children right at home.

Hula Hoop

Loosen up those hips, get your groove on, and let it all hang out with a hula hoop, another great idea for a lazy afternoon. Take turns, and have contests to see who can last the longest; and for an even better time, do it to music and see if everyone can hula to the beat.

Playing with the Dog

Rolling around with the dog, believe it or not, can be great exercise—and better yet, it also gets the dog exercising. Playing with the dog can be a full-body workout and requires little planning or preparation. It can just happen whenever. This way, every member of the family, human or not, gets in on the wellness and fun.

Limbo Dance

Maybe it's our tropical blood, but we love a limbo dance in our house. Remember that limbo should not just be relegated to cruise ship vacations in the Caribbean—actually it's great to play right at home. We love it because it has a sort of yoga aspect to it, through the deep back bend; and it also always sparks a festive, party-like atmosphere.

Dancing

Dancing is to the body what laughing is to the soul. Again, maybe it is our Latin blood, but there's no doubt about it: we are a family of dancers. There is nothing like letting loose and feeling the music along with the people you love most and feel most comfortable with. Dancing and music have the capacity to take you to a place you can't get to any other way. It relieves tension in the most magical way. It brings happiness. Dancing is the equivalent of letting your character out to play. Not only does this activity (which can happen anywhere, anytime) engage the body but it also asks the spirit to abandon inhibi-

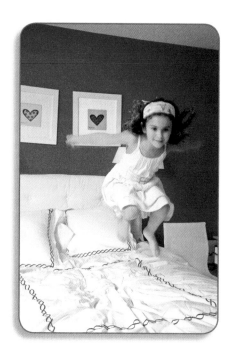

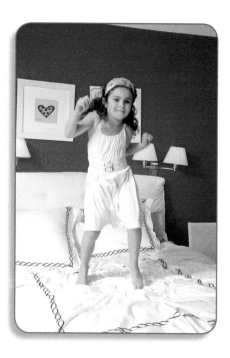

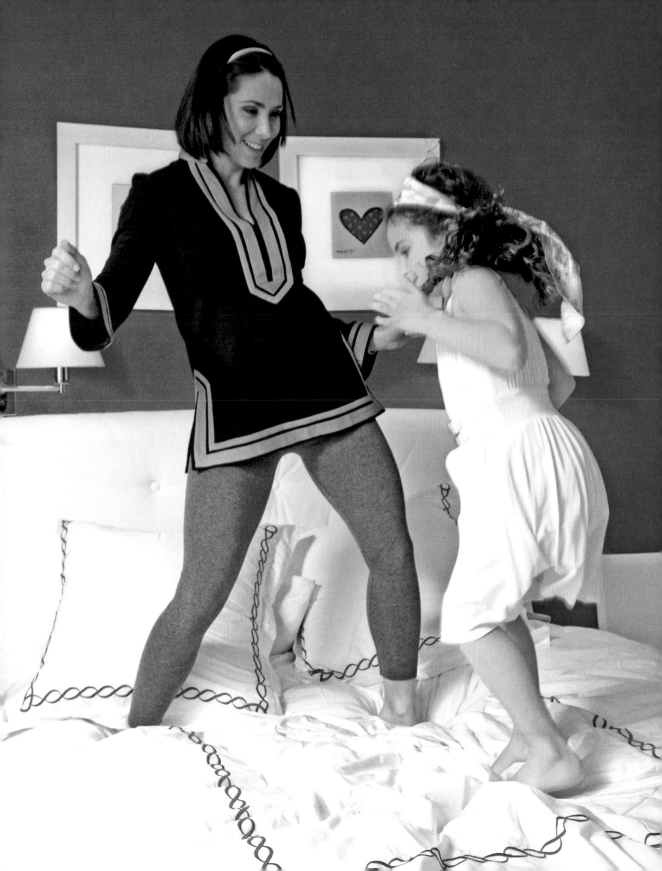

tion and strut its stuff. When you're in a bad mood, stressed out, overwhelmed, even a bit tired—there is nothing like a good old dance to jolt the system with a shot of pure energy.

Pillow Fight

All's fair in love and war—*pillow fight* war, that is. Pillow fights are wonderful because for the most part they are totally safe and simultaneously demand that the participants give it their all to reign supreme. And when you do give it your all, a pillow fight can engage the entire body. Best of all is the fact that this is a perfect nighttime activity, or something to spark on a lazy Sunday, when everyone's just lolling around at home.

King of the Bed

This one holds a special place in our family, and it is essentially the game of "conquering" the bed, by somehow keeping all the other players off. You do this by using pillows as shields for yourself and the rest of your body to try to push the other players off—making sure to be careful and not play too rough. Our kids love it, and when their friends come over to our house, they all want to play too. King of the Bed is basically a next-level pillow fight, taking the competition for dominion ever more seriously. King of the Bed is a game of control and power, and in our house, it's one of those things that can happen every single night without anyone ever getting bored. This activity has become a Posada staple.

Board Games

Board games can be the perfect answer to a late Saturday, after the sun has set, before the evening kicks in. Recently we had a snow day and ended up having to stay in the house for about ten hours—well, we played about ten hours of board games, all kinds of different educational games, mind games, and creativity games. We had some dominoes around, so we used them to play multiplication games with our son, Jorge Luis, and with our daughter, Paulina, who's younger, we practiced addition. Using most of the games that we had around

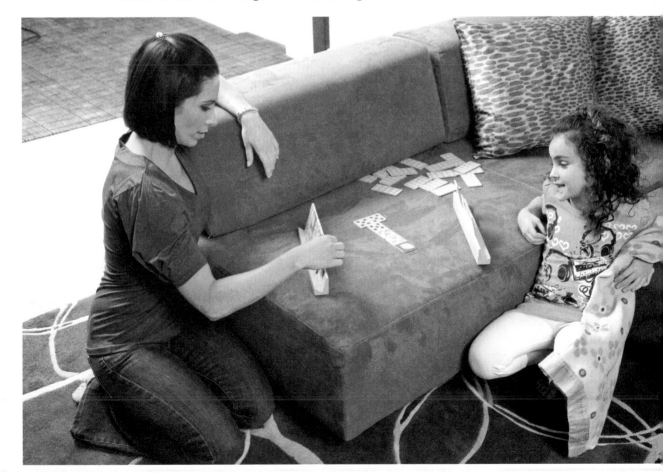

the house, we managed to have a completely full, dynamic day.

Board games stimulate the mind and encourage group dynamics and accountability. As a group, prepare some healthy snacks and hunker down with one of your favorite games. Keep score, play by the rules, and call people on their mistakes—and remember that sitting around to play a board game with your family can be just as nourishing as a bike ride in the park.

One of the games we love is Life, very obviously because it teaches you about life. It makes you think about things like college, occupation, house, mortgage, marriage, and so many other fundamental aspects of being an adult in the world. We also love Sorry! and Scrabble Junior.

Wii Fit

Wii Fit is where we bend our rules on video games, perhaps because this is the one video game that also bends the body. With yoga, balance games, strength training, and aerobics, this interactive virtual game makes the viability of full-spectrum exercise possible for everyone right from your very own living room.

Karaoke

Sing it loud, and sing it proud. One of the best gifts you can give to your kids is a karaoke machine, and one of the best things you can do with your family is plug in and belt out some of your favorite songs. This activity is not only a lot of fun it

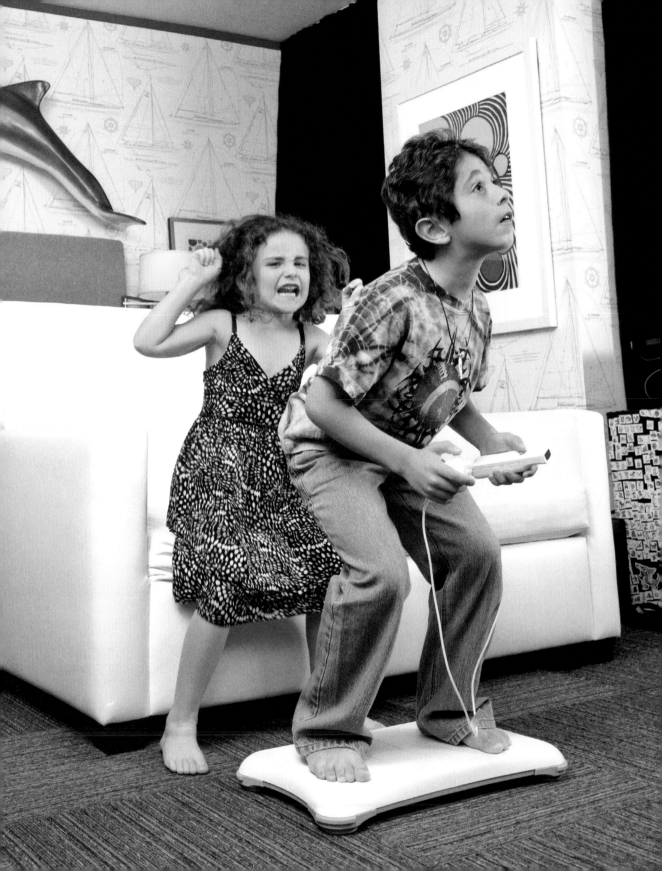

works on people's sense of confidence and comfort levels. But most of all, karaoke is just a consistently reliable rip-roaring good time.

Turn Home into Gym

The beauty of this one is that is forces you to reacquaint yourself with your home and become more resourceful about how you approach its many uses—but only if you are crafty enough to do so. Turning your home into a gym shows your kids (and yourself!) that you do not require anything fancy to get your exercise. A kitchen chair can become the designated place for triceps dips, for example; an outdoor ledge can become a place where people (those who can) do pull-ups; and the spot under the sofa can be where people sneak their toes to do a set of sit-ups.

You should also be resourceful about your own grown-up workout time. If you can afford a treadmill or stationary bike for use at home, we highly recommend you get them and take every chance you can to use them. When kids are napping or playing with friends, it is the perfect time to hop on the bike for a quick half hour. Take advantage, and keep it easy, by having the access in the comfort of your own home.

Swinging Blanket with Song

We used to do this one with our kids when they were babies, and they absolutely adored it. All it means is that the child lies in a blanket (make sure it's heavy enough), and the parents each grab a side of the blanket (with both hands, of course) and swing the kid, as if they're on some kind of metric hammock that runs on the power of human love. Oh, and we sing a song while we do it. If you are the parents of little kids, just give it a whirl. Do it for as long as you can, and you'll see that in time they will simply be too heavy for the game; so it's nice to enjoy this old favorite while they're small and easy to hoist.

Family Talent Show

The family talent show is one of the most amazing ways to get everyone's creativity flowing and keep everyone entertained the whole time. It asks each member to focus on their own "thing," and calls on the spirit of performance and sharing to make the whole thing feel "real." The talent show is a way to loosen people up, especially the more timid ones. Remember, if you gently nudge them to open up at home, they are more likely to do so out in the world. Our daughter, Paulina, for example, loves to play her mini electric guitar and improvise rock numbers for us; our son, Jorge Luis, loves to tell jokes. Everyone has something they love to do—encourage them to look for it and own it with all their hearts. You never know what kinds of talents you are planting the seeds of in the future.

Coloring

Coloring is a great way to get your kids relating to color and playing with art. We find that when our kids color, there is a

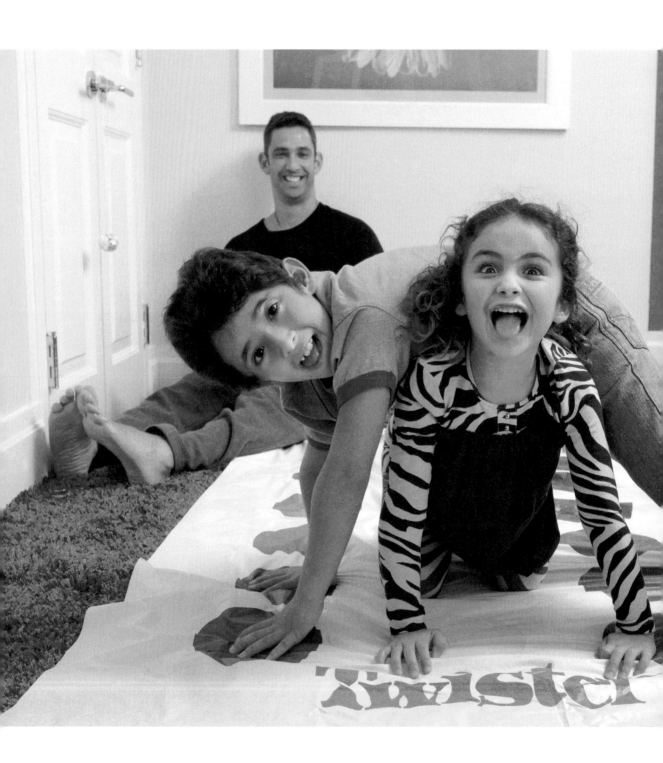

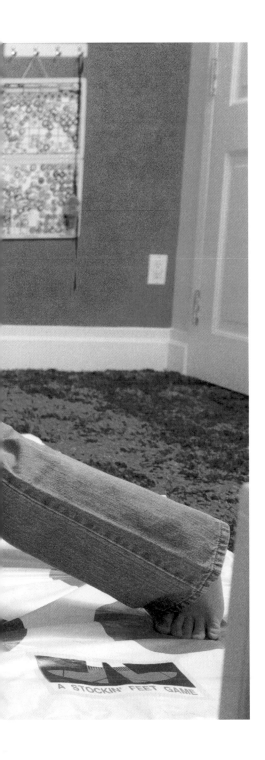

calm about them; it is somehow therapeutic for them. In any case, it's a great activity for a rainy or snowy day, and portable enough to take anywhere on the road.

Play-Doh

Play-Doh is a great and relatively mess-free way to get your kids thinking about the fine art of sculpture. It asks them to use every shred of their imagination to shape the world as they see it, making for potentially rich sessions of stimulation and creativity.

Twister

This is the board game that doesn't let you get bored—because *you* are the pawn, and your body is your weapon. This one is a great icebreaker, especially if the kids are grumpy and not really in the mood for anything in particular, or if your spouse is cranky and you feel like lightening the vibe in the house. Twister brings the kid out of everyone and gets the body moving and stretching.

Ping-Pong

We fully understand that not everyone has a Ping-Pong table. But maybe one year, assuming you have the space for it, you decide it is the perfect Christmas gift. Why not? Ping-Pong is that good old-fashioned "rec room" activity, and isn't that exactly the kind of atmosphere you want to engender at home? Have Ping-Pong championships; play singles or doubles; or just see how long you can keep volleying the ball. Many family centers and community centers have Ping-Pong tables, and make note that when you travel, most hotels will also likely have a Ping-Pong table. It's the kind of game everyone can play, from small children to grandparents alike.

Meditation

If you believe the practice of meditation should be reserved for monks in mountain retreats, think again. The art of doing nothing is actually quite beneficial for everyone, including children, whose quick minds are always running and could stand a moment of total stillness. Teaching them to stop and zero in on what's happening inside is an important tool that you can impart to them early in their lives. Don't be intimidated by the word *meditation*. Instead, think of it as a simple closing of the eyes, accompanied by long, deep, luxurious breaths. Your only job is to do nothing, except to follow the path of your breath.

Try this three times a week with your kids, and you'll notice just how much calmer and centered they will seem. It might help you to know that in India, schoolchildren are actually taught to master the skill of meditation.

Remember that many of these activities, whether they take place indoors or outdoors, are not only perfectly suited for you to play, enjoy, and practice at home but also happen to be ideal for scenarios where the family is traveling, or for families on a budget. In either case, the games work because they do not require much, and because they have that universal quality that makes them viable anywhere.

Many of these suggestions for games are also great to have on hand when you are dealing with little girls who have no interest in sports and would rather spend their time working on arts and crafts or playing with dolls. That's perfectly fine: simply incorporate their crafts and dolls into the more active pursuit, such as the obstacle course, for example, which is a favorite among the more creative kids, who are stimulated by spatial, colorful things. You can create missions and tasks such as running across the room and painting something on the other end, and then running back and unscrambling some words on a sheet of paper, as part of a mental challenge. Feel free to really mix it up.

Do not force your kid to have an athletic character if it is simply not there, but *do* work with the ideas we have presented to find ways of keeping even the least athletic kid active and strong.

GENERAL ACTIVITIES FOR SMALL CHILDREN AND TODDLERS

Toddlers and preschoolers need plenty of time to just run around free and play at will—so playgrounds, parks, and the beach are all great places for kids at this age. Here are great ways to keep physical activity fun no matter where you are with the little munchkins. These also happen to be great ideas for pregnant mommies who need to move but also need to take it easy.

- Use a large, soft ball to start teaching the basics of throwing, catching, and kicking a ball.

- Play games involving rolling, skipping, hopping, and chasing.

- Invent some silly walks with your child, such as running like a monkey or hopping like a bunny.

- Encourage tricycle riding, and play with push toys such as trucks and doll strollers.

- Pack away the stroller and opt to walk to the library, park, or shops.

- Chase things like butterflies, dragonflies, and bubbles.

- Play different kinds of music to encourage creative dancing and a sense of rhythm.

ACTIVITIES WRAP-UP

We know that many of these suggestions and ideas were not new to many of you, and that's OK. The point was not necessarily to introduce you to these concepts—but more to remind you that they all exist, and likewise to encourage you to introduce them to your own children, given the modern world that they inhabit, where a lot of the staples and classics are getting lost amid the unstoppable hustle of our ever-evolving technological advancement. Do not assume that your kids are familiar with all of these activities and games just because you are; in fact, assume just the opposite, and use your role as parents to spark interest and stimulation whenever you can, however you can. We offer this list in the hopes of getting you excited and with the goal of giving you brainstorming material and off-the-cuff tips.

The real agenda was to tickle the part of your mind that knew about all of these amazing games and ideas, the part that lingers in the memory of your own youth, reminding you that *any* activity with your kids is better than nothing at all. Our mission is simple: to gently urge you away from a life of idleness and toxicity, toward a more mobile, physical lifestyle where you and your children can jointly thrive. Needless to say, though we encourage as much family time as possible, we also encourage you to get your kids involved in activities with other kids, such as sports leagues or courses at the local Y. Find venues where your kids can shine, and push them to do so. Remember that at the end of it all, they will be better armed to perform well out in the world, now that you have been on your own family mission of fitness.

Final Pep Talk from Our Hearts

So there you have it, in black and white, the secret to our success and the base of our formula, which as you now know boils down to one primary thing: *family*. If we have not made it clear enough, we would like to reemphasize that nothing on this planet matters more to us than the inner sanctum of our family, with our children at the epicenter of this sacred bond. If we maintain this truth, which we always do, then we must stand solidly by the value and import of raising our children to become the healthiest, strongest, most balanced adults they can be—an endeavor that we know will not happen all on its own. It requires our directed, dedicated work, discipline, effort, and the kind of conscious awareness that we have been discussing throughout the pages of this book.

We sincerely believe that the pursuit of fitness and proper nutrition is fundamentally about self-love, which is not to be confused with vanity. When you truly love yourself from the bottom of your heart and soul—which has absolutely nothing to do with vanity—*you are good to yourself,* and that is what true wellness is all about. This is the lesson that we hope you will be inspired to teach your children, so that they continue to tread on their individual paths in this world as their most confident, capable selves, poised to fulfill every single one of their dreams and aspirations.

Teach them that the secrets to a quality life are actually quite simple, and that by just honoring the seasons and paying attention to Mother Nature's built-in cues, they can enjoy this amazing universe in all of its natural glory, and savor its many delicious foods at just the right moment. Teach them to pay attention to the details, to those amazing flashes of magic, like rainbows, shooting stars, and sun showers; to the mysteries of the night, like crickets and wind; and to the sounds of babbling brooks in the crevices of mountains, or massive waves exploding on a white-sand beach. Teach them about the natural synchronicity of enjoying fish and seafood when you're sitting near the beach; the perfection of sipping hot chicken soup out of a mug on a cold and rainy day; or the joy of a frosty frozen yogurt cone on a hot summer day. Show them that there is a right time and a right place for everything, and that with food and likewise with fitness, you can always take your elemental cues from nature itself. This way, eating moves out of the realm of being something we do to quell cravings, and into the natural order of things, to partake of when the time and place are just right.

Teach them that all of this wonder and amazement is possible all the time, especially if the family commits to fostering a recreational life that includes the outdoors, activity, stimulation, and creativity, which you will now be armed to do, having gone through this book. Make sure your family also understands the nature of *commitment,* and what it means to make up your mind about something. Use the power of the group to constantly strengthen the might of that commitment. Talk to them about discipline and the need for consistency, and how success does not happen overnight but one little burst of effort at a time. Remember that what you are aiming to do here is reshape the way each family member understands their individual role in the potential for their own future, and to help them see the simple ways people can be their most effective and positive selves in the world.

If the prospect of transforming your family's bad habits into good ones is entirely overwhelming and seemingly impossible to you, try to shift your attitude to a "one-change-a-time" kind of an approach. Start by making small changes, such as implementing vegetarian nights or planning a weekly outing to a local park. Consider investing in bikes for the whole family or plan a weekend trip that includes hiking and kayaking. Take your hula hoop and a flying disk next time you go to the beach. Play lots of music in your house, so the mood and collective energy are always up. Make it a point to smile with your children, and radiate unstoppable love with as much of yourself as you possibly can. Give your family members compliments more often, and instead of getting grumpy about something someone did, ask them to go with you on a walk or a bike ride. These are just a few of so many little modifications that will start to tweak your old family routine, and you will soon see that each one will be another layer explored toward your ultimate goal of cultivating a happy, healthy, and active family.

Easier said than done, we know. We also know very well that life can get hectic and busy and everything can seem to get uncontrollably frenetic, without enough time, money, or energy to ever do anything, much less worry about family fitness. But this is exactly the mind-set that we all need to start moving away from, understanding that by incorporating fitness, we will in fact alleviate the nervous hustle of our daily lives, because we will be naturally better fit, mentally and physically, to navigate through them.

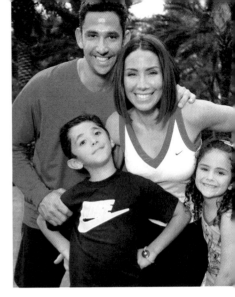

Furthermore, our committing to doing all of this as a group takes it to an even higher level, because by infusing our entire effort with the collective energy of determination and motivation, we give the goal more weight and load it with more personal meaning. It becomes *our* goal, a common goal, one with significant purpose and very obvious benefits. And, most critically, it keeps us all together. In the end, it is this ultimate purpose that we seek as a family: to spend our precious time productively, actively, meaningfully—but most important, to spend it *together*.

Despite our own very busy lives, we have dedicated ourselves entirely to our children, and hold as our highest priority their consistent well-being. In our experience, the best way we ensure this is always to supply them with the knowledge and resources to be the best they can be right now, and for the rest of their lives to come. We encourage you to refer to this book, to use it as a guide, to use it as a motivator, to use it in any way you need, in order to light the proverbial fire under your seat, and *start making the changes that will make your family shine*. Life is short, and if it has taught us anything through our experiences, good and bad, that we have endured as a group, it is that the power of this blessed little collective is all we really need.

Family Progress Chart

	Physical Activities	Vegetables Consumed	Fruits Consumed
Week 1 Dad's weight: _____ Mom's weight: _____			
Week 2 Dad's weight: _____ Mom's weight: _____			
Week 3 Dad's weight: _____ Mom's weight: _____			
Week 4 Dad's weight: _____ Mom's weight: _____			
Week 5 Dad's weight: _____ Mom's weight: _____			
Week 6 Dad's weight: _____ Mom's weight: _____			
Week 7 Dad's weight: _____ Mom's weight: _____			
Week 8 Dad's weight: _____ Mom's weight: _____			

Water Consumed	Lean Protein Consumed	Challenge of the Week	Notes

ACKNOWLEDGMENTS

We would like to thank our children, Jorge Luis and Paulina, for helping us when we needed the calm and quiet to write; and for collaborating with us like a pair of little adults, working so hard to complete photo shoots; Johanna Castillo at Atria Books, for believing in us; Natalia Ferrer, our close friend who always helps to make our ideas into reality; the New York Yankees for allowing us to use their facilities and always supporting us as a family; and finally, deep gratitude to all the coaches and trainers that taught us everything we know about being athletes and the art of pushing your body and mind to the limit.

For a complete resource list, please visit www.fithometeam.com.

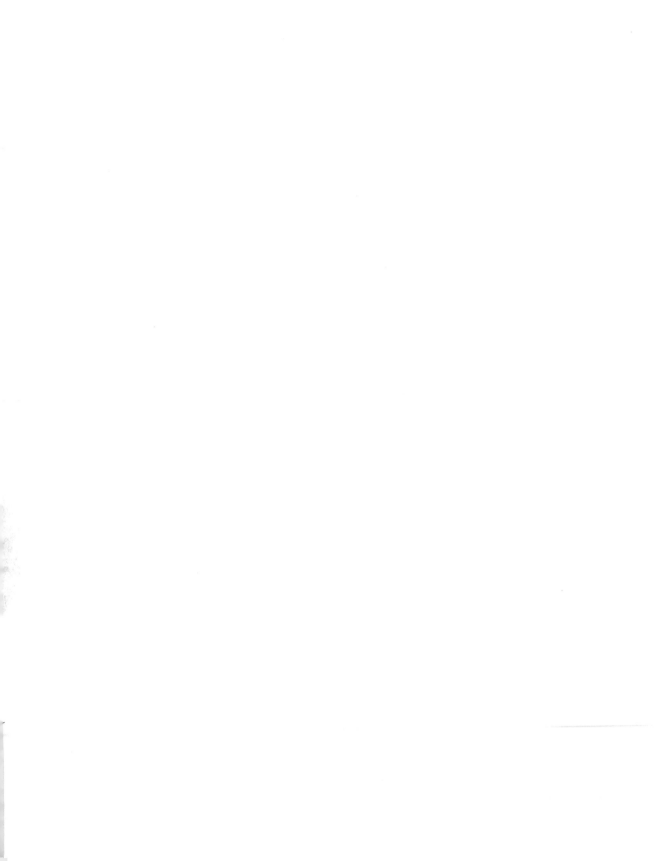